V A C C I N E S

THIS BOOK COULD REMOVE THE FEAR OF CHILDHOOD ILLNESS

Also by Trevor Gunn:

'Comparing Natural Immunity with Vaccination'
ISBN: 978-0-9554678-0-2
www.vaccinesideeffects.co.uk

'SomaWisdom – The Science of Health & Healing'
ISBN: 978-0-9566914-0-8
www.somawisdom.org

Trevor Gunn BSc Hons LH RSHom
Medical Biochemist Registered and Practising Homeopath
www.homeopathy-soh.org

Currently At:
The Dyke Road Natural Health Clinic, Brighton, UK
www.dykeroadclinic.co.uk
And
The Japan Royal Academy of Homeopathy, London, UK
www.rah-uk.com

Trevor Gunn BSc Hons LCH RSHom
Can be available for talks & presentations
Please contact:
enquiries@trevorgunn.com
Trevor has presented in the UK, Ireland, Japan, Egypt,
Lebanon, Iceland, Croatia and on National TV and Radio

Acknowledgements

I gratefully acknowledge the support and patience from all of my dear family members, Jodie, Mirelle, Leon and Ylana in assisting the creative environment for me to work. I should also like to thank Phil Akilade, Colin Grant and Jamie Taylor in the arduous task of editing and encouraging my volumes of writing. Last but not least I extend my humble gratitude to all patients, students and participants of my lectures; they have equally given as much as I have received from the many experts I have encountered.

CONTENTS

CONTENTS

PREFACE

What if you were made to believe that 'most' of your fellow citizens were potential murderers, intent on killing you and your loved ones? That without adequate protection, almost all encounters in your daily life would be a threat to your existence, and that each and every one of these people would lay in wait for the first available opportunity to enact deeds of violence. You would then of course take precautions.

It would be irresponsible not to, where possible, you would isolate your children, only venture out when protected; bullet proof jackets, alarms, GPS tracking, fire-arms, but could you ever feel safe?

To make matters worse we would be constantly reminded that our enemies are perpetually evolving, adapting for the sole purpose of bypassing our defences to execute their destruction, and that if they got one child they could more easily learn to get another. And so of course our only hope of survival would lie in the continual development of more and more potent weapons and defence mechanisms.

This is the biological scenario given to us by vaccine promoters, where the risks of protection are a necessary evil for us all, because of an inevitable and intimate contact with a dangerous biological environment. A place where mistakes can have fatal consequences and with even the best 'protection' there are grave but unavoidable risks. A precarious existence on a constantly evolving planet where our defences will eventually become outdated, and so a world where very few people can ever really feel safe.

But what if we found out that our vaccine promoters were wrong about the nature of our world, that scientists and biology had long since moved on. Would vaccine promoters change their strategy, would they own up to the true nature of this world, would they overplay the risks of disease, would they fully admit to the dangers of vaccines, and in the real world, would the risks of vaccines be acceptable?

This book shows us how certain sectors of the medical community have misinterpreted the fundamental nature of disease, adopting strategies that are unfortunately blinding us to the ease in which serious disease can be avoided and increased health can be attained. The unnecessary fear of disease has led us to accept seemingly protective vaccines with a desperation that has left us oblivious to their unacceptable consequences.

To make choices about vaccines we need to understand their true side-effects, we need to be able to balance those against the real risks of disease, and then with knowledge of viable alternatives, we are then able to make effective health choices. With all of the necessary information, without censorship from those with vested interests, we are able to do just that.

The information presented in this book goes a long way towards satisfying those needs, as well as acknowledging the emotions involved in the decision making process, the emotions exploited by the selling of drugs, vaccines or in fact any commercial commodity. With information and awareness we may then be empowered to be in control of our health and to once again feel safe in our world.

CHAPTER ONE

1 Why is vaccination such an emotive and controversial issue?

1.1 Safety issues

Mass vaccination policies have been generally recognized as being responsible for safely and effectively, reducing and eradicating diseases world-wide, the first mass smallpox vaccine campaign was introduced to the UK in 1840.

Yet in recent years vaccines have become repeatedly embroiled in controversy, especially concerning their safety. In the 1990's a mumps vaccine found to be causing encephalitis was later withdrawn, vaccines repeated linked to autism, mercury in vaccines associated with neurological damage, polio vaccine containing SV40 cancer virus, flu vaccines predisposing patients to Alzheimer's, plus the known side-effects of allergies, autoimmune disease, paralysis and even cot death to name but a few. And in addition to the spectre of vaccine damage there are now many researchers daring to question the purported effectiveness of vaccines against a backdrop of vaccine criticism that has existed since their inception.

The following lists the known side-effects of vaccines that you will find stated on vaccine packages, the acknowledged adverse effects amount to a catalogue of potential medical disasters, vaccine producers know that harmful effects can occur:

> *Redness, swelling, soreness or tenderness at the vaccine site, mild to moderate fever, tiredness, drowsiness, poor appetite,*

headache, nausea, vomiting, mild rash, seizure (jerking or staring), non-stop crying - for 3 hours or more, high fever, swelling of the lymph nodes (lymphadenopathy), inflammation of the parotid gland (a salivary gland near the ear), low platelet count (thrombocytopenia) which can cause a bleeding disorder, serious allergic reaction (breathing difficulty, shock), pneumonia, pain and stiffness in the joints (mostly in teenage or adult women), chronic and acute arthritis, nerve inflammation, long-term seizures, severe paralytic illness (Guillain-Barré Syndrome), coma, or lowered consciousness, brain inflammation (encephalitis), permanent brain damage and death.

There may appear to be some controversy as to whether vaccines can cause for example autism, however in the USA Hannah Poling was awarded damages from a settlement reached in 2007, disclosed in March 2008, a case of autism where United States government lawyers agreed that it was triggered by childhood vaccinations, more recently 2009 Bailey Banks awarded damages for acute brain damage involving autistic spectrum disorder from his MMR vaccination. It is of course not an issue of whether vaccines cause autism but in how many.

1.2 The Fear of infectious disease

1.2.1 Often unduly hyped and marketed to promote a particular policy using technical jargon and statistics; Swine flu, bird flu, Sars.

The motivating force to risk the potential damage of the vaccine is of course the benefit in avoiding more dangerous infectious diseases. The vaccine therefore has to be effective, the disease needs to be prevalent and equally the disease needs to be dangerous enough to warrant administering a potentially harmful vaccine.

Overplaying the risk of disease could therefore be a marketing strategy for vaccine promoters; the whole issue is of course an immensely fear laden one. Would vaccine manufacturers use such tactics?

Dr Marc Girard was commissioned as an expert medical witness by the French Judge residing over compensation claims for the families of those that died soon after receiving the Hepatitis B vaccine in France. Dr Marc Girard spent 1000's of hours on the subject with access to dozens of confidential documents, unfortunately what he found, in simple terms, was that the WHO had grossly overplayed the dangers of the actual disease and profoundly underplayed the dangers of the Hepatitis B vaccine. Dr Marc Girard had unearthed an efficient web of coercion exerted by the commercial manufacturers of the vaccine under the auspices of the WHO:

> *"It is blatant that in the promotion of the hepatitis B vaccination, the WHO has never been more than a screen for an undue commercial promotion, in particular via the Viral Hepatitis Prevention Board (VHPB), created, sponsored and infiltrated by the manufacturers (Scrip n° 2288, p. 22).*

Further observations revealed that these were not isolated incidences, in his research Dr Girard was then able to see a parallel with another disease making the headlines at that time, 'avian flu' otherwise known as 'bird flu'.

> *It is quite easy to reconstruct that, under the lame pretext of increasing the manufacturing potential, the manufacturers managed to induce the WHO's experts to recommend flu vaccination, whereas it is plain that this immunization would have no protecting effect against avian flu.*
>
> *In both situations, the trick was the same: to create a false alarm…*

In addition the more recent handling of the swine flu pandemic of 2009 had all the hallmarks of the previous campaigns, with overt fear mongering and drive for vaccine sales. Predictably disease forecasts were found to be grossly exaggerated whilst pharmaceutical companies made a fortune in vaccine sales, and by the spring of 2010 the Council of Europe launched an investigation into whether the World Health Organization (WHO) "faked" the swine flu pandemic to boost profits for vaccine manufacturers. The inquiry, held in Strasbourg, France, vindicates a worldwide movement of insiders, experts and elected officials who accuse the United Nations organization of misleading the world into buying millions of unnecessary vaccines.

The opinion given by Dr. Wolfgang Wodarg, an epidemiologist who formerly led the health committee for the Council of Europe, is that the World Health Organisation changed their criteria for defining pandemic levels to boost vaccine sales.

> "There is no other explanation for what happened. Which reasons could lead to those [WHO] decisions? I don't find any other explanation. It's not for health. And who profits? Why else would you change the definition?"

Paul Flynn (Vice Chairman - Council of Europe Health Committee)

> "...The world has been subjected to a stunt for their own greedy interests of the pharmaceutical companies"

1.3 Feeling that we are not given all the information to be able to make informed decisions as parents

Many parents feel they need more information in which to make informed decisions but find it difficult to obtain anything other than the standard vaccine promotional blurb. As an example of attempted censorship the parenting magazine ABC printed a pro-vaccine article in which I was also asked to write a response, to show the other-side of the vaccine debate. The magazine was distributed through various outlets in the South of England; public and private venues, businesses that had taken advertising in the magazine and various NHS buildings. However, after publishing the edition with both the pro and opposing views it was in fact removed from all NHS outlets. So rather than respond to vaccine criticisms the 'powers that be' decided it was more useful to simply remove the magazine, as far as they could, from the public domain.

Although the difficulty of accessing information is a reality for many, even more worrying is the fact that researchers themselves appear to be stifled in their work:

Dr Michel Odent working at the Primal Health Research Centre in London found a link between whooping cough vaccine and asthma; a report of which was published in The Journal of the American Medical Association in 1994. What astounded Dr Odent was the refusal of health authorities and other researchers to look into the effects of whooping cough vaccine in relation to the increase in asthma. In a public debate in London in which I was also a panel member, he expressed frustration at the authorities in looking at every other issue, dust, pollution, home furnishings…"even the colour of the carpet" but in no way are they willing to look at the possibility of vaccine damage.

Paul Shattock at the Autism research Unit, at Sunderland University is similarly critical. In his research, he's found that approximately 10% of autism cases that he has investigated is caused by the MMR vaccine, but he states that he is not allowed to research those cases that are due to the vaccine and the University will not publicly endorse those findings, even though they are willing to stand by his findings in other areas of research regarding autism.

Carol Stott, Department of Psychiatry, Cambridge University studied a cohort of children believed to be damaged by the MMR vaccine and found a significant link between the onset of autistic symptoms and the administration of MMR vaccine. The heads of the department at Cambridge University were similarly convinced of the link, suggesting, as Carol Stott did, that it required further study. However because GlaxoSmithKline (a manufacturer of MMR vaccine) funds research for Cambridge University Psychiatry department, Carol was told further research in that area would be like ..."sawing off the branch that holds us up." Carol Stott had to abandon the research.

1.3.1 In addition many scientists are actually surprised at the lack of knowledge that vaccine promoters have about their own vaccine components and their effects:

What are the agreed safe levels of aluminium in vaccines?
Until recently there were no upper safety levels set for environmental exposure, but the European Food Safety Association has newly recommended an upper level in dietary intake of 1mg per kg of body weight per week (22 May 2008). Acknowledging that 99.9% to 99.7% will be excreted through the gut and never enter the blood and internal systems of the body, but this absorption level can increase by as much as ten fold if other factors are present in the diet that aid assimilation.

Therefore the recommendation allows that a possible 3% of the upper safety limit could be absorbed into the body. A 6 month old child, maximum body weight 10 kg, would therefore have an upper safety limit of 3% of 10 mg aluminium per week having access to the internal body which is a **weekly maximum** of **0.3mg** yet a single injection can contain 2.5 times that at **0.85mg**, with many children with much more reduced body weights receiving that in one day.

Are these levels in vaccines safe? It seems that the upper limits recommended for vaccines have been guessed and assigned by**... we don't know who...** as revealed by the transcripts from the National Vaccine Program Office Workshop on Aluminium in Vaccines, May 2000.

Dr. Gerber, National Institute of Health in fact asks the question:

"... the standard of 0.85 milligrams of aluminium per dose set forth in the Code of Federal Regulations, can you tell us where that came from and how that was determined? "

Dr. Baylor appears qualified to answer that question, he is: Acting Deputy Director of the Office Of Vaccine Research and Review, and Associate Director for Regulatory Policy at the Centre for Biological Evaluation of Research at FDA... however his answer is somewhat revealing:

"Unfortunately, I could not. I mean, we have been trying to figure that out. We have been trying to figure that out as far as going back in the historical records and determining how they came up with that and going back to the preamble to the regulation. We just have been unsuccessful with that but we are still trying to figure that out."

So we are injecting neurotoxins into our children and adults, and the vaccine community does not know what levels are safe, but do in fact appear to be guessing at doses...this of course isn't science. As Dr. Martin Myers, Director of the National Vaccine Program Office, Department of Health and Human Services recognises and states in the same meeting:

"Perhaps the most important thing that I took away from the last meeting was that those of us who deal with vaccines have really very little applicable background with metals and toxicological research."

1.3.2 Research scientists get scared of vaccines

Neuroscientist Chris Shaw and a four scientist team from the University of British Columbia and Louisiana State University, conducted studies to test the possible impact of vaccines in the emergence of Gulf War Syndrome.

Shaw is most surprised that the research for his paper hadn't been done before. After 20 weeks studying vaccinated mice, the team found statistically significant increases in anxiety (38 percent); memory deficits (41 times the errors as in the sample group); and an allergic skin reaction (20 percent).

> *"For 80 years, doctors have injected patients with aluminium hydroxide, an adjuvant that stimulates immune response. This is suspicious, either this [link] is known by industry and it was never made public, or industry was never made to do these studies by Health Canada. I'm not sure which is scarier."*

> *"No one in my lab wants to get vaccinated," he said. "This totally creeped us out. We weren't out there to poke holes in vaccines. But all of a sudden, oh my God-we've got neuron death!"*

> *"To me, that calls for better testing, not blind faith."*

1.4 Many parents when ask the question about safety are often dismissed by the medical profession

Many parents will have first hand experience of emotional responses from doctors if they choose to question vaccines or even simply ask for information especially if they express concern of vaccine safety and effectiveness. Parents' reports of their children's negative reactions to vaccines although very likely, are often met with disbelief by their own doctors and consequently disregarded.

> *"I was in support of vaccines and was comfortable with the fact that there is a national database that records "all" vaccine reactions so they can see trends and such – which is the info I got from my doctor.*

Then, my daughter had a reaction to a vaccine at 18 months old. **It was horrifying to watch** *her body swell for three days and not be able to do anything (Benadryl slowed the swelling, but couldn't reverse it until three days had passed). I knew there were risks to vaccines, but it had seemed that the benefits outweighed the risks. I could have accepted that.*

I was not prepared for the reaction of the medical community. **My doctor's office refused to admit it was a reaction** *– even while she was swelling! They were concerned about the swelling, asked me if I knew how it started, then, when I mentioned that I suspected the vaccine they sent me home and said I was imagining things. A few hours later she had to go to the ER. Later I took her to* **an allergist who confirmed that it was a reaction***. He told me that a lot of people react to the 3rd DTaP shot – even if they've been fine before. Still, he encouraged me to continue getting all the shots except for the last DTaP.*

No one ever reported any of this to the national database.

My pediatrician pressured me to get more shots for my kids, but I refused. I've recently found out my **kids' medical records falsely state that my kids DID get additional vaccines.**

My daughter had been ahead on speech milestones at the time of the reaction, from that date (October) to the following July, she only learned 8 new words, and **her language development froze. We've done three years of therapy now and she is in special education***.*

1.5 Lots of the available information can appear confusing and incomplete

In the UK there has been much controversy over the findings of Dr Andrew Wakefield linking the use of MMR vaccine with regressive autism, a potentially severe and debilitating, behavioural and emotional condition. Consequently confidence in the vaccine has diminished considerably among the general public and the government health authorities have been at pains to try and restore faith in the vaccine. In 2001 the UK health authority publicised a report of a study conducted in Finland, citing this as proof that the MMR vaccine does not cause autism. However, closer examination of this study only serves to illustrate the problems associated with the governments prejudice and tunnel vision when assessing adverse effects of vaccines. The report appeared convincing, involving 1.8 million children over a 14-year period finding no link between MMR vaccine and autism. There were however major limitations to the study:

> The study relied on voluntary notifications of adverse effects, in which experts agree, at best; pick up 10% of incidents.
> Secondly the reactions that were being looked for; fits, allergies, neurological disorders, rheumatoid arthritis and diabetes – did not include autism or any symptoms associated with it.
> Thirdly the reported adverse reactions concentrated on a three-week period after vaccination and would therefore miss the slow appearance of symptoms associated with regressive autism.

The study was therefore completely inadequate in its ability to assess the incidence of regressive autism.

This Finnish report was not based on a study of the effects of MMR, it was not an independent research project on the effects of MMR on the human physiology, but a look at the reports sent in to the local health authorities. Reports that were not looking for autism or any symptoms associated with autism, in a time-frame outside of the normal appearance of symptoms, therefore highly unlikely to find any symptoms of autism associated with the use of MMR vaccine.

Yet the government cited this as scientific evidence that MMR does not cause autism. If we then take into account the fact that the report was supported by a grant from Merck & Co, USA, a producer of MMR vaccine we see that there have been inherent conflict of interest issues and that this was not an independent study. Furthermore the subsequent documents, aimed at restoring public confidence in MMR, distributed to doctors in the UK was authored by Mike Watson medical director of Aventis Pasteur also a manufacturer of MMR vaccine. This is of course worse than inadequate and appears to indicate a level of intentional neglect amounting to deceit.

1.6 Lots of vested interest riding on its continued use

Vaccine production is a billion dollar industry; most are sold to governments and health authorities around the world. The market, unlike most other pharmaceutical products, consists of virtually everyone on the planet that can tolerate and afford vaccines. Unlike most other drug treatments, aimed at a small section of the population that have a particular illness, vaccines are given to the healthy, the potential for profits are huge. The following analysis of the promotion of flu vaccine illustrates the nature of the 'vaccine' as a product for profit, the methods used to coerce users i.e. the general public, are shrouded in the language of public health information, but are of course sales techniques.

Peter Doshi, "Viral Marketing: The Selling of the Flu Vaccine." March 2006.

> "The influenza vaccine is a national industry, with President Bush asking Congress to fund a $7.1 billion flu preparedness plan".

> There is a strategy for selling flu shots. 2004 National Influenza Vaccine Summit, Glen Nowak of CDC explained how certain messages generate buzz and drive demand.

The recipe, as Nowak revealed, relies on creating "concern, anxiety, and worry" its main ingredient, in other words, is fear.

Government officials and health experts are instructed to: "Predict dire outcomes."

2002 focus group, the CDC determined that death statistics were "eye catching and motivating." Participants in the study believed "20,000 deaths was compelling, frightening" and "should be part of the headline."
In 2003, the agency began announcing that the number of Americans killed each year by flu had surged to 36,000, an 80 percent increase that is now widely reported.

Among all flu-prevention messages in the news during the week of 9/21/03, according to Nowak's presentation, "Flu kills 36,000 per year" appeared second most often, just behind "Doctors recommend/urge flu shot."

But the 36,000 figure is actually a measure of "flu-associated" fatalities, almost exclusively among the elderly and infirm, whose deaths from other illnesses the CDC thinks might not have occurred without the flu but not caused by flu. Records show that only 1,400 deaths a year are attributed to flu.

1.7 What impact on wider pharma industry if the vaccine story is discredited?

If vaccines are discredited, many of the underlying principles of disease and immunity may come into question, consequently other approaches to health-care would appear more appropriate. The problems of vaccines could lead to a major overhaul of the current medical approaches to treatment and disease prevention, thereby affecting sales of other pharmaceutical drugs as well as vaccines in general. There is of course a massive financial commitment to the current pharmaceutical method, but equally a considerable mental and emotional investment in an orthodox medical philosophy that does in fact form the basis of many peoples' lives and belief systems.

There are the obvious ramifications of financial liability to drug companies and governments should vaccines be admitted as the cause of damage to children and adults, but there may be more widespread implications in terms of a wider re-assessment of health-care intervention. This could lead to a much reduced role of the pharmaceutical industry and medical orthodoxy, with patient choices leading them away from a drug approach to health-care.

There is already a decline in confidence in a pharmaceutical system of health intervention, with the results of drug-use never meeting the exaggerated claims of big pharma sales in addition to the prospect of an ever increasing number of dangerous side-effects. Patients are becoming more aware of the life-style choices that affect their health and are therefore more knowledgeable of the simple and safer alternatives to drug intervention. The outcome of vaccine safety and effectiveness studies has financial, political and emotional repercussions, all of which heavily influences the information that is readily available to the general public.

1.8 Parents that question vaccines find themselves under attack.

Although there is a lot of vested interest in vaccines, most members of the public that question their safety and effectiveness find that they receive the greatest criticism and emotional attacks not from the experts but from their more immediate acquaintances, family and friends. Those deciding not to vaccinate have often carried out an extensive review of the available scientific literature and would have by necessity looked at both sides of the argument, yet they find themselves accused of being ignorant, irresponsible and irrational in their approach.

There are of course many people that have chosen to vaccinate and have never felt the need to question the advice of their health authorities and their doctors. Many of these people feel threatened when they come across those that question the safety and effectiveness of vaccines; these emotions may be based on the fear of increased disease from the unvaccinated, but given that vaccines protect these people this would appear to be a mute point. There is of course the defense of vaccines on the basis that they reduce the levels of disease in the population and therefore protects even those that are not vaccinated. We shall deal with this issue in more detail later, however this is not usually the basis for most people's emotional defense of vaccines.

There may be many reasons for the hypersensitive reactions of people on both sides of the debate; however it is interesting to note that many of those vehemently defending vaccines know very little about vaccines, immunity or disease, in my experience the scientists that know the most are far more measured in their responses. We have unfortunately a large number of what we can call 'non-expert experts'; scientists, health practitioners, journalists and members of the public. This is not a statement of their ability to reason or understand the issues, but a term defining those that have not read the research and/or have very little experience in health care yet are vociferous in their condemnation of those that choose not to vaccinate.

On the face of it there is a lot of research that demonstrates the safety and effectiveness of vaccines, but there are ubiquitous problems with most of that research, as many scientists know. Therefore reading the summaries, abstracts and conclusions to these studies will not give you the details that one needs to assess the value of that research. This in itself is common, most people, doctors included, do not read the entirety of research studies:

> *"Some doctors are scientists—just as some politicians are scientists—but most are not...*

If doctors are not scientists then it seems odd to supply them, as medical journals do, with a steady stream of original scientific studies. Teachers and social workers are not sent original research. Nurses are sent some, but are they simply aping the illogical ways of doctors?

The inevitable consequence is that most readers of medical journals don't read the original articles. They may scan the abstract, but it's the rarest of beasts who reads an article from beginning to end, critically appraising it as he or she goes. Indeed, most doctors are incapable of critically appraising an article. They have never been trained to do so."

Doctors are not scientists. BMJ 2004; 328 (19 June)

The critique of vaccines cannot be addressed by simply regurgitating the standard view, the critique needs to be studied and specifically responded to; virtually all of the emotional defense of vaccines thrown at members of the questioning public is at best rhetorical but unfortunately of little substance.

CHAPTER TWO

2 Do vaccine promoters understand the illnesses that vaccines are supposed to prevent?

In order to understand the basis of the widely differing opinions about the safety and effectiveness of vaccines we shall need to assess the impact of vaccines on the health of individuals and of the general population, as well as the theoretical foundation of its use. We shall be looking at both the detail and the overview; the detail as elucidated by biological sciences and the overview as often revealed by the evidence of holistic medicine. Disciplines that were once considered poles apart are actually converging, revealing a picture of health and disease that is in fact congruent to both.

In assessing the role of vaccines in health care, as indeed any medical procedure, we need to assess its possible benefit versus potential side-effects. The benefit of the vaccine in terms of the reduction in incidence of disease; - does the procedure reduce the numbers of people contracting the illness and therefore will it make you less likely to become ill. In addition there is the benefit of the vaccine in terms of any reduction in severity of disease; - if you were to be vaccinated and still contract the illness, will the vaccine reduce the severity of the symptoms of illness and ultimately make you less likely to die from the illness. These potential benefits would then need to be weighed against any potential damage that the procedure of vaccinating could cause.

On the face of it, the vaccine debate seems to be confined to issues of rare side-effects, the issue of overall value, however, appears to be undeniable, a 'fait accompli', vaccines in the eyes of many are of unquestionable merit, their virtues extolled by most of the medical profession. A procedure believed to have been safely and successfully used for decades, instrumental in the modern medicine's triumph over disease, a belief shared by professionals and public alike. But of course not all health care practitioners are in agreement; in fact, an opposing view is just as vehemently upheld by a growing number of orthodox scientists, doctors as well as alternative therapists.

In making an assessment of the value of vaccines it would seem logical to just get the facts; obtain the necessary statistical details and all the relevant information on vaccines, carry out the tests, conduct appropriate trials and choose the best way forward. However, as many of us are aware, much of the information does appear contradictory, with health care practitioners holding vastly differing beliefs. In such a climate of disagreement between our so-called experts, how are members of the public able to reach conclusions and make effective health choices? In such situations, in order to make sense of apparently contradictory 'facts', we are often in need of a little more overview.

A flat earth continued to be the accepted doctrine long after the evidence was available to demonstrate that the world was in fact round and we would have found ample evidence demonstrating both points of view. We can now envisage how it is possible to produce more and more evidence showing us what appeared to be the perfectly logical truth that the earth was flat, yet still be 'incorrect' in the bigger picture. In order to fully understand the issue of our planet we needed to expand our view of the earth to appreciate how it could be round and at the same time essentially flat in our local experience of the ground upon which we walk and upon which we build. It was vital to have greater overview, from that point we could develop our understanding of the motion of bodies towards the centre of the earth to realise why material objects always fall towards the ground i.e. towards the centre of the earth and do not in fact fall off of the edge of a round earth and so appear to fall to the floor wherever we are, as though the earth was indeed flat.

Similarly in making an assessment of vaccines we need to understand in simple terms current vaccine theory and then of course the bigger picture in terms of the underlying premises and their historical context, are there other more encompassing theories of health and illness that enable us to understand the full impact of vaccines and our experts current contradictions? We need to evaluate the consequences of vaccines on the cellular level as well as their effect on the whole person and the greater community, whilst taking into account the impact of other factors on health and illness. We will then be more able to understand how differences in opinion have arisen, make a more measured assessment of the impact of vaccines and more importantly judge whether it is a procedure we would wish for ourselves and for those in our care.

2.1 Vaccines: The underlying assumptions.

2.1.1 Vaccines & Infectious disease

Vaccines have been created to produce immunity against infectious diseases, diseases that are considered to be potentially life threatening or significantly debilitating to warrant medical intervention. Vaccines were developed to prevent illness and were therefore initially produced on the basis of certain assumptions as to how these illnesses are contracted and on further notions regarding the best way to create immunity to these illnesses. We shall start by looking at the foundation of these ideas whereupon we can then start to make our own predictions regarding the consequences of various forms of medical intervention including vaccination.

2.1.2 Immunity and Infectious disease

Both the general public and medical professionals are in general agreement about the mechanisms of infectious disease, including the basic principles of how to avoid and treat these illnesses. Most people believe that microbes, (bacteria, viruses, fungus etc.), invade us from the outside, thus causing the infectious illnesses; with some microbes being more virulent than others and consequently more dangerous than others.

We have also been lead to believe that we are open to infection at any time and although we can do a certain amount to stay healthy, some microbes can affect and kill even healthy people.

Therefore we are told that the best way to avoid infectious illness is to actually develop immunity to that illness. It is thought that immunity can be obtained by two methods:

1. Naturally, by exposure to the microbe and therefore developing symptoms of the illness, the condition itself would provide life-long immunity.
2. Or acquired, artificial immunity, through the use of vaccines.

According to method one, for example contracting 'measles' naturally and developing symptoms of measles, including the development of the measles rash etc, this would confer life-long immunity to the measles microbe. By our method two, artificial immunity, the use of measles vaccine, such as with MMR, would hopefully create artificially acquired immunity to the measles microbe with little or no symptoms of illness.

It is generally believed that natural immunity carries a certain amount of unquantifiable risk; it is possible that you could suffer any one of the many serious 'side-effects' known as 'adverse effects' from the illness, but we could not say for sure which, if any, would happen to you.

Blindness, deafness, brain damage or even death could happen as a result of measles infection. Some infectious illnesses themselves for example paralytic poliomyelitis are far more serious than typical measles. It is therefore acknowledged, by many people within the orthodox medical community, that vaccine-induced immunity is potentially safer than naturally acquired immunity.

In addition to the above ideas of infectious disease and immunity, there is another fundamental concept inherent within the system of orthodox medicine and that is the concept of 'malfunction'.

Human beings are, supposedly, like sophisticated machines and from time to time things will go wrong, and when they do, we produce symptoms of illness. Just as a machine that starts to malfunction needing the expert engineer to fix it, our symptoms of illness show us that we need fixing by the doctor, we will need to be put right. Like a household appliance that no longer works, a leaking pump, a blown fuse, a broken belt, the only way it can function normally again, is if it is fixed and if it is not fixed, things can only get worse.

In such human instances of malfunction, we are also likely to deteriorate and therefore in the case of an illness, this can ultimately lead to our death. Therefore medical expertise will also involve sophisticated means of screening for early signs of malfunction, with the development of diagnostic technology able to detect increasingly smaller deviations from the norm. Then with the use of pharmaceutical drug intervention the ability to put things right before they deteriorate further. Best of all, medical experts will aim to develop preventatives such as vaccines, able to put things right, almost imperceptibly, before anything even starts to go wrong.

2.2 Infectious disease a historical perspective

A brief look at our medical history will give some insight into how we have arrived at our current concepts of infectious disease and immunity, thereby providing a basis for understanding how we have arrived at our conventional approach to medicine. A medical approach largely dominated by mechanical models of health and illness, that although extensive in detail, often lack overview and context and therefore lacking the required meaning and significance necessary in the understanding of how and why illnesses occur.

2.2.1 Germ theory - what 'lies' beneath. The historical and underlying concepts of infectious disease - Pasteur & Béchamp

A cursory glance at medical history will reveal the name of Louis Pasteur, born 1822 in Dole, France, his name forever immortalised on a day-to-day basis in 'pasteurised' milk – named in his honour. As described in most conventional medical history texts, he has been credited with having transformed medicine, his contributions being that:

> ➢ He showed that airborne microbes were the cause of disease.
> ➢ He built on the work of Edward Jenner and helped to develop more vaccines.

However, a closer look at historical records will reveal otherwise, the basis of germ theory with the discovery of microbes was in fact originated by other scientists and their conclusions regarding the causes of illness were very different from that of Pasteur. Germ theory itself was postulated years before Pasteur had claimed it to be his own and so having copied the work of others Pasteur took several more wrong turns before developing theories of germs and infectious disease that were more acceptable in the 19th century. Theories that were more acceptable to the general public, medical community and government, many of whom had an agenda and were looking for a hero to champion the cause, and that hero was to be Louis Pasteur.

In the West, medical theory with regards to infectious illness was actually consolidated with the work of Antoine Béchamp when he took up the study of fermentation (1854). He was a contemporary of Pasteur and to place their beliefs in context we shall look at the perennial question asked by scientists and philosophers both then and now:

> ➢ What were the origins of the universe, life and effectively ourselves, how and when did it all begin?

At the time of Pasteur and Béchamp, approaches to this question could generally be divided into two:

> One theory was that the substance of the universe was at some time created out of nothing and that 'creation out of nothing' was either spontaneous or due to the work of some kind of omnipotent God and that this phenomena could happen at anytime. It was used to explain the mechanism of some diseases and the appearance of simple life forms in decayed substances etc.

> The other perspective being, that life had evolved out of substance that was always present, an evolutionary point of view. That is to say, the stuff of the universe, the planet and life on earth had always existed in some way, shape or form and had slowly evolved into forms of ever increasing complexity to what we see of life today. Life was not and could not be created spontaneously out of nothing. This was often considered to be the more 'scientific' view.

In the 19th century at the time of Béchamp and Pasteur, the commonly held doctrine, was that of 'substance out of nothing' and was called "spontaneous generation", a view supported by many scientists including Pasteur.

However, Béchamp not content to ascribe certain life processes to the theory of spontaneous generation studied three biochemical phenomena:

1. Sepsis
2. Fermentation
3. Grape diseases.

He demonstrated that there were small organisms involved in all of these processes, organisms that he later called 'microzymas', (effectively what we now call microbes). These microbes actually lived within the material of the substances of the above examples, digesting nutrients and producing waste products, existing like tiny animals in an ecosystem of food, water, shelter and toxic waste. He also demonstrated how they could be transferred through the air to contaminate other samples. Although this had been suggested before, Béchamp was the first to demonstrate this through scientific experimentation.

At this point he had not distinguished the various forms of microbes from each other i.e. fungal cells, bacteria, viruses, etc, but was however the first recorded scientist to demonstrate the effects of microbes, showing how they were able to exist and therefore interact within the larger 'host' organism and how their by-products would have subsequent effects in their host.

In the examples given:

> **Sepsis** – when a wound becomes septic producing pus: Bacteria and white blood cells destroy and digest dead cells and foreign debris at the site of an injury and the waste products of this cellular digestion forms the green pus seen at the site of a septic wound.
> **Fermentation** – sugar solution into alcohol: The small organisms are yeast cells which would feed off sugar, and the waste product of this sugar digestion is alcohol, thereby it appeared that under certain conditions sugar solution would turn into alcohol. Whereas in fact alcohol is being produced by the digestion of sugar by yeast cells.
> **The grape disease** studied by Béchamp was caused by certain microbes on the skin of the grapes which digest the grape juice extract and excrete waste products that affect the health of the grapevine and more importantly the quality of wine produced.

In 1857 Béchamp had irrefutably demonstrated the activity of these microbes and the concept of this microbial activity was therefore used to explain the mechanisms of the above processes. This was 'the' giant step forward in our understanding of microbes in fermentation and microbial diseases. Prior to Béchamp, scientists including Pasteur, explained fermentation as a simple 'spontaneous' chemical transformation without involving microbes.

The deficiency of Pasteur's knowledge as compared to Béchamp is also apparent when we consider other experiments of Béchamp. Béchamp was able to demonstrate the activity of microbes in mixtures that had previously no microbes present; Béchamp concluded that these microbes were able to enter via the passage of air. However other scientists including Pasteur said this was due to microbes 'spontaneously' emerging. Pasteur's theories and experiments are clearly documented to have been years behind Béchamp.

In fact in 1859, two years after Béchamp had conducted his experiments and one year after publishing the conclusions of those experiments, Pasteur was still referring to the activity of microbe fermentation as "taking birth spontaneously" and therefore not acknowledging the passage of microbes in the air. Pasteur lacked the conceptual framework of Béchamp that would give him the ability to design experiments that could demonstrate the activity of microbes, yet it was Pasteur that had laid claim to having first discovered and demonstrated the existence of microbes in the air.

Pasteur carried out very little original experimentation and has been widely acknowledged as having plagiarised the work of Béchamp. In the 1940's book by R.B. Pearson originally published under the title "Pasteur, Plagiarist, Imposter", Pearson describes a meeting of research scientists at the Sorbonne University in Paris, Nov 22, 1861. Here Pasteur had to admit to knowledge of Béchamp's work whilst previously claiming credit for the proof of microbe theories as his own.

RB Pearson, in "Pasteur, Plagiarist, Imposter".

Dr M.L. Leverson MD PhD MA an American Physician, discovered some of professor Béchamp's writings in New York and immediately realised they had been published before Pasteur. He travelled to France to meet Béchamp and in a lecture entitled Pasteur, the Plagiarist, 1911 outlined Béchamp's claim to priority and added the charge that Pasteur had deliberately faked an important paper.

He said in part:

"Pasteur's plagiarisms of the discoveries of Béchamp, and of Béchamp's collaborators, run through the whole of Pasteur's life and work…"
"Finding how readily the 'men of science' of his day accepted his fairy tales, published in the Annales de Chimie et de Physique 3rd S., Vol. LVIII, there is a section entitled Production of Yeast in a Medium Formed of Sugar, of a Salt of Ammonia and Phosphates.
The real, though not confessed, object of the paper was to cause it to be believed that he, and not Béchamp, was the first to produce a 'ferment' in a fermentative medium without albuminoid matter. Now mark, I pray you, what I say – the alleged experiment described in the memoir was a fake – purely and simply a fake. Yeast cannot be produced under the conditions of that section! If those of my hearers or any physician having some knowledge of physiological chemistry will take the pains to read this section of Pasteur's memoir with attention, he will see for himself that yeast cannot be so produced, and he can prove it by making the experiment as described."

"…I cannot but believe that the exposure I am making of Pasteur's ignorance and dishonesty will lead to a serious overhauling of all his work."

Dr Leverson goes on to say…

"From the outline I have now given you, you may form some idea of the ignorance of the man who, for more than thirty years, official medicine has been worshipping as a little god. But this is only a small part of the mischief perpetrated. Instead of making progress in therapeutics during the past thirty or forty years, medicine – outside surgery – has fearfully retrograded, and the medical profession today is, in my judgement, in a more degraded condition than ever before in it's history."

However this admission to Béchamp in the company of other researchers that Béchamp had already proved the existence of microbes did not stop his continued self-proclaiming as the discoverer of the activity of microbes.

Paul de Kruif in 'Microbe Hunters' speaks admirably of Pasteur…

"Pasteur invented an experiment that was – so far as one can tell from careful search through records – really his own. It was a grand experiment, a semi-public experiment, an experiment that meant rushing across France in trains, it was a test in which he had to slither on glaciers"

An experiment carried out in 1864 as recorded in the 14th edition of the Encyclopaedia Britannica showing how Pasteur proved the existence of… "organisms (microbes) with which ordinary air was impregnated".

However, it was a phenomena **already proved by Béchamp, seven years earlier, in 1857**.

It was in fact from the ideas of Béchamp that eventually lead Pasteur in the 1870's to conclude that:

➢ Microbes would cause illness after having infected the person via the passage of those microbes through the air.
➢ Each specific microbe would cause an illness that was unique to that microbe.

This was the "<u>Germ Theory of Disease</u>" discovered first… supposedly by Pasteur as claimed by …Pasteur.

According to the principles of 'germ theory', diseases were caused by the entry of microbes into the body from an external source, and were called 'infectious diseases', each specific microbe causing its own specific disease. Therefore if somebody has measles illness, a measles microbe from the environment must have infected him or her and this microbe could be the only cause of measles. Another individual with for example chickenpox would therefore have to have been infected by a separate chickenpox microbe and this microbe is only capable of producing chickenpox illness and not measles.

This germ theory of disease, as with the theory of the passage of microbes in the air was again something that Pasteur claimed to be his own, even though in fact "germ theory" had been postulated long before. A fairly comprehensive summary of germ theory was postulated by M.A. Plenciz in 1762, 100 years before Pasteur had popularised it as having been his own, Plenciz stated:

> *"There was a special organism by which each infectious disease was produced, that microbes were capable of reproduction outside of the body, and that they might be conveyed from place to place by air".*

More recently, in 1993, according to Gerald Geison of Princeton University, examination of Pasteur's laboratory notebooks reveals that there were astonishing discrepancies between his notes and published writings, Geison states:

> *"Pasteur lied about the numbers involved in trials and about the production of the anthrax vaccine later used in a public trial, all of which helped both him and later his Pasteur Institute in Paris to become extremely wealthy and famous".*

Sylvie Simon writes of the works of Dr Philippe Decourt, Ethyl Douglas Hume, G Gerald Geison, Xavier Raspail, Daniel Raichvarg and others; from probing many authenticated research papers they reveal that Pasteur claimed for himself discoveries made by others and with the help of accomplices he doctored unfavourable experimental results and tyrannically refused to discuss them.

The drama of a 12-year-old child who died as a consequence of the vaccination revealed the dishonesty of Pasteur and his colleagues. On 16 October the child died. An inquiry under Professor Brouardel sought the cause but the lofty, titled, professor was a friend of Pasteur. Brouardel, in agreement with Roux, decided to falsify the evidence before the inquiry. In Les Vérités Indésirables - Le Cas Pasteur, Philippe Decourt records that it was a matter of avoiding official acknowledgement of a failure that would entail, according to Brouardel, "an immediate step backwards in the progress of science" as well as dishonour to Pasteur.

Pasteur vigorously opposed Henry Toussaint's theories and practices, which he said were ineffective and dangerous. To prove that his vaccine was better he agreed a protocol of experiments that would come to fruition on 28 August 1881 at Pouilly-le-Fort, near Melun. On the appointed day Pasteur confided to his associates that he would not use his own vaccine but Toussaint's. Who today is aware that the Pouilly le Fort experiment was no more than a hoax?

2.2.2 Germs, friend or foe?

In any event, plagiarism and historical inaccuracies aside, Pasteur had popularised the germ theory of disease and in so doing placed the responsibility of illness on the infecting microbe, the 'germ'. The germ was said to enter the body from an external source, causing illness in the unsuspecting individual and was therefore said to be the primary cause of infectious illness.

It is worth noting at this point that Pasteur had never managed to prove or demonstrate that these illnesses were actually caused by infecting microbes, i.e. microbes that were not already present within the system. The idea that illness was caused by a microbe infecting the human body from the external environment was just that …an 'idea'.

Pasteur's theories suggest that if you have a pathogenic microbe (one associated with a disease) that you did not have before, then it must have come from the outside and because microbes do not change form, it could not have been produced from other microbes already within the person. This is known as 'monomorphism', one definitive unchanging physical form, for each type of microbe. Therefore, once within the body, these microbes are able to multiply and the fear is that they could equally be given to others, thus spreading disease.

Béchamp on the other hand, went on to show that the microbes responsible for the diseases that he observed were actually already present before the initiation of the disease, he therefore deduced that the most important factor was the nature of the host material, i.e. the constituents of the bodily fluids and tissues upon which the microbes grew and multiplied. According to Béchamp it is the medium in which the microbes live and feed that determine whether the microbe produced substances that would enhance the health of the individual or whether they produce toxins that would exacerbate symptoms of disease. He also demonstrated that health conferring or benign microbes could therefore change into pathogenic microbes according to the nature of the patient's cellular environment.

Indeed Béchamp, and other scientists that followed, concluded that the micro- organisms involved in disease processes were in fact cleaning up the internal environment; they do not live off healthy living tissue but diseased and dead tissue.

The ability of microbes to change form is termed pleomorphism and was an inherent part of Béchamp's observations and teachings; this was to be confirmed later in the 20th century by other scientists Dr Gunther Enderlein, Dr Rife, Dr Gaston Naessens, Dr Wilhelm Reich with microscopic techniques able to use live tissue samples.

Most observations of cells are conducted with light microscopes, the samples are usually thinly sliced and/or stained so that the various components can be seen against the background, but this means that the samples have to be killed, preserved and fixed in a suitable material.

However scientists working with live blood samples, use what is called 'dark-field' or 'dark-phase' microscopy, a different lighting technique is employed where the samples are not stained or killed and they are able to observe microbes changing into these different forms according to the nature of their environment; the more acidic, the less oxygenated and the more polluted the bodily fluid, the more we find associated microbes. As acidity and toxicity levels increases and oxygen concentrations decrease these microbes grow larger and accumulate protein reserves as an adaptation to their environment and practitioners are able to remedy diseases by addressing the conditions that create internal toxicity.

Researchers using dark field microscopy are able to diagnose illness by observing these changes in microbes that are normally resident in each person, and are able to remedy diseases by addressing the conditions that create these imbalances.

These facts have been largely ignored by the present orthodoxy, mainly because they appear to undermine their own perspective and approach to treating illness. Orthodox interpretations tend to think of microbes as static elements unable to change form, known as monomorphism, and that pathogenic microbes are either present or not and that healthy human blood is sterile and therefore free of microbes. Therefore the way to deal with the presence of microbes in illness is to simply kill them.

However, modern microbiology has in fact refuted all of the original assumptions of the monomorphic tradition, even though those doctrines still dominate our clinical medicine. In orthodox medical texts pleomorphic organisms are now acknowledged to exist, for example the rickettsia organisms involved in typhus. In addition, as published in the Journal of Clinical Microbiology, August 16 2002, conventional microbiological methods, have demonstrated the existence of populations of pleomorphic bacteria in <u>healthy</u> human blood.

Even from orthodox interpretations of illness, there are also known disease phenomena that would suggest a soil theory takes precedence. The theory of a 'carrier of disease' makes an allowance for the fact that all individuals carry potentially disease-causing microbes and yet do not have symptoms of illness but are in fact perfectly healthy; polio viruses, haemophilus influenza bacteria, meningococcal bacteria are associated with life threatening conditions, many are present within all of us yet we experience no symptoms of disease.

It is also known that a carrier can subsequently become ill from the previously present, though apparently dormant, microbe, in spite of which the medical establishment rarely questions the nature of this change. If carriers can become unwell from resident microbes, then a medical approach to treatment must involve an understanding of how that person became susceptible to the germ, it is therefore likely that killing the germ would leave the susceptibility unaltered.

For example in Australia with modern disease notification records and where families are more apt to live in isolation on their vast farmlands, children have been documented as having contracted chickenpox and other childhood illnesses when there has been no contact with anybody for months yet alone with anyone with chickenpox that could have 'given' them the illness. The standard incubation periods, in which the microbe can be harboured within an individual before symptoms are manifest, are usually estimated at around two to four weeks maximum. It is clear that these microbes exist within us for much longer periods and therefore the onset of symptoms may <u>not</u> be caused by the infecting microbe, but by a change in the internal environment of the patient. Once these changes have occurred the patient becomes susceptible to illness and opportunistic microbes proliferate.

In the NHS Public Health Network newsletter, 16th May 2002 Birmingham UK, under the heading 'Predisposing factors' there were concerns as to the reported cases of measles, none of the normal factors that could have caused the outbreak appeared to exist. The report stated that:

> None of the reported cases of measles were immuno-suppressed i.e. none were taking immune suppressive medication.
> None had a history of overseas travel.
> None had a case of measles in their family or had contact with a known case.

This highlights the possibility that some individuals may develop measles from within; not necessarily caught from external sources. Almost 150 years after the soil theory of Béchamp, reports of pathogenic microbes that exist within the body become news worthy.

2.2.3 Seeing things differently to see different things

Therefore even though there appears to be only a subtle difference, the concept of disease according to Béchamp takes on a radically different flavour to that of Pasteur's germ theory. As far as Béchamp is concerned, microbes are present all the time, they are in and around us, and it seems there needs to be a significant change to the substances in which they grow, in order for them to multiply and therefore become associated with symptoms of disease. Diet, toxins, hormones, acidity, emotions, hydration, etc all influence the environment in which microbes live and grow in the human body and this environment, we shall call the 'soil' of the microbe. Like the soil of farmland, the nature of the earth and the climate around the earth, this determines what can be grown there.

From this perspective the substances in which the microbes grow, the "soil", takes on the greater significance, and not the presence or absence of these microbes, this we shall therefore refer to as Béchamp's "soil" theory of disease.

Béchamp's 'soil theory' relies upon the understanding that:

> There are changes in the proportions of existing microbes that can be associated with symptoms of disease, for example small numbers of fungal cells are tolerated within the body but if you kill off large numbers of bacteria, with for example antibiotics, a greater proportion of fungal cells will dominate and create illnesses associated with fungus.

> Microbes can change from one related type to another - from health conferring microbes to microbes associated with disease. This type of change is what is known as 'pleomorphism'.

> In addition to this there are also bacteria that produce certain healthy substances in certain circumstances but produce toxins if forced to live in other conditions for example in oxygen depleted environments.

If, as according to Béchamp, microbes do behave in this way, then of course illness cannot be avoided simply by avoiding contact with microbes in the external environment, even though they can be transferred from one person to another, they can equally be produced within. Similarly, killing microbes associated with disease without addressing the conditions that are creating them will not stop more of them from being produced from the many millions of microbes already within the body.

2.2.4 Florence Nightingale

A very interesting counter-argument to germ theory comes from an unlikely source, Florence Nightingale (1820-1910), 'the lady with the lamp'. Famous for her contribution to nursing during the Crimean war, she gained many insights into the nature of disease. Medical history tells of a rather subsidiary role for nurses, although highly commendable, nursing has nevertheless been portrayed as rather secondary to the function of 'real doctors'. Florence Nightingale was however more outspoken than we have been generally led to believe.

The voice of Pasteur may have been immortalised and Florence Nightingale relatively obscured, however, it appears as though she had some strong opinions regarding the theories of infectious disease.

Florence Nightingale did in fact endorse a perspective of infectious illness akin to that of Béchamp and published a counter-argument to the germ theory, in favour of a "soil theory" of disease. She acknowledges the influence of the human condition on the microbes, where microbes change from one type to another and therefore potentially pathogenic microbes are always present within an individual. Published over **17 years before Pasteur's claim to have originated the germ theory of disease**, this is further evidence that 'germ theory' was in fact common knowledge within the medical fraternity long before Pasteur had claimed to originate the idea himself.

Florence Nightingale…

"Is it not living in a continual mistake to look upon disease as we do now, as separate entities which must exist, like cats and dogs, instead of looking upon them as the reactions of kindly nature against the conditions against which we have placed ourselves?

I was brought up by scientific men to believe that smallpox was a thing of which there was once a specimen in the world, which went on propagating itself in a perpetual chain of descent, just as much as there was a first dog or pair of dogs, and that smallpox would not begin itself anymore than a new dog would begin without there having been a parent dog.

Since then I have seen with my eyes and smelt with my nose smallpox growing up in first specimens, either in closed rooms or overcrowded wards where it could not by any possibility have been "caught" but must have begun. Nay, more, I have seen diseases begin, grow and pass into one another. Now dogs do not pass into cats. I have seen for instance, with a little overcrowding, continued fever grow up, and with a little more, typhoid fever, and with little more, typhus, and all in the same ward or hut.

For diseases, as all experience shows, are adjectives not noun substances. The specific disease doctrine is the grand refuge of weak, uncultured, unstable minds, such as now rule in the medical profession. **There are no specific diseases, there are only specific disease conditions.**"

Using the analogy of cats and dogs Florence Nightingale states that if illnesses are defined by microbes and these microbes are monomorphic, i.e. could not change from one type to another, then they could not begin out of nothing and one could not be created from the other, a cat could not be created from a dog and neither of them could be created without a parent cat or dog. However her experience shows that illnesses do behave like this, illnesses appear to start and change from one type to another simply by changing the conditions of the patient.

Illnesses, according to Florence Nightingale, are approximate descriptions of the nature of the patient and how they react to the conditions in which they live. She categorically states that illness is therefore not a 'thing', what she calls a noun substance and cannot be defined by the nature of an unchanging infecting microbe, but disease is determined by the nature of the patient and their diseased conditions. A doctrine that was however viewed as erroneous by the medical establishment and even today according to the Florence Nightingale Museum Trust, London, they quote:

> *"Like her friend, the public health reformer Edwin Chadwick, Florence Nightingale believed that infection arose spontaneously in dirty and poorly ventilated places. This mistaken belief nevertheless led to improvements in hygiene and healthier living and working environments."*

It is of course interesting, that her 'mistaken belief' lead to improved health.

Historical anecdote paints a rather interesting picture of the ultimate beliefs of Pasteur, Lionel Dole (1965) in his writings on the history of vaccination:

"Most people cherish their delusions even more than their other ailments. As Thomas Edison was fond of saying: 'There is no expedient to which Man will not resort to avoid the hard work of thinking.'

The germ theory and the idea that 'germs can be conquered by vaccines', was one of the most greedily grasped of all such expedients. It was so much more modern and scientific than the fuddyduddy idea of mending our ways or atoning for past errors. Man wants to believe that the maladies he brings upon himself are all due to those terrible germs, which, being unable to sue for libel, are the ideal scapegoats. What a tremendous debt we owe to Louis Pasteur, the Microbe Man!

And yet **Pasteur himself, at the end of his life, was quoted by his old friend, Prof. Renon,** who attended him in his final illness, as having said:

"Bernard was right. The germ is nothing. The soil is everything."

It cannot be believed that this final scientific utterance of Pasteur's is not authentic, but it is not inscribed on the wall of his tomb, nor have we ever heard it quoted on the radio."

However, Béchamp's theories have since been relegated to obscurity, often described as "the lost chapter of biology", and concomitantly the theories of Pasteur have dominated, until perhaps, a more recent resurrection.

2.3 Why germ theory and why Pasteur?

Within the human body, there are trillions of microbes; they live in a 'symbiotic' relationship with each one of us. A symbiotic relationship is one where the microbe and the host live in <u>mutual benefit</u>; in fact they are often dependent on each other for survival, (as distinct from a parasitic relationship wherein a parasite lives at the expense of the host. Here of course the host does not benefit but often supports the parasite to the detriment of itself).

Microbes within the human body are necessary for your health

Dr. Gibson, Food Microbial Sciences Unit, at The University of Reading, UK in 1996 states that …

> …" *There is much variability in bacterial numbers and populations between the stomach small intestine and colon. In comparison to other regions of the gastrointestinal tract, the human colon is an extremely densely populated microbial ecosystem - with the resident microbes representing around 95% of all cells in the body. The large gut flora is now accepted as playing a major role in both human pathogenesis and health - with the colon being the body's most metabolically active organ. Through diet, the composition of this microbial ecosystem can be influenced such that micro organisms which are benign or health promoting can he stimulated.*"

These microbes produce essential nutrients, aid in digestion and keep down levels of other potentially harmful microbes; however, these same microbes that are essential for health could equally become pathogenic (cause symptoms of disease) if conditions were to change; conditions that are influenced by, nutrition, toxins, enzyme levels, acidity, hormone levels, physical injury, emotional trauma, etc.

Therefore, many 'infections' can be more accurately described as 'imbalances' or even seen as positive symptoms of 'rebalancing' and are the result of the bodily conditions supporting these microbes. The microbes would have almost always been present prior to the onset of illness. Therefore it appears that microbes are the result of disease conditions and not the primary cause. REMEMBER here the context of this statement of microbes; the alternative to germ theory is that although microbes are associated with illness they do not create the diseased condition of the patient in the first place; the diseased condition came first and produced the conditions for the microbes to grow.

We must also remember that different microbes have their home in specific parts of the body and that true infection i.e. movement of microbes already within the body, to other parts of the body, can occur as a result of injury or disease. For example the movement of bacteria from colon to blood and then to the nervous system, as a result of the breakdown of the immune system and digestive membranes, could lead to septicaemia and meningitis. These microbes did not newly infect the patient but are necessary and existing microbes that are always present but have been allowed to invade the interior of the patient as a 'result' of disease.

2.3.1 An idea whose time had come.

"I have had my results for a long time: but I do not yet know how I am to arrive at them."

Karl Friedrich Gauss

Quite why Pasteur's views dominated so strongly has been fertile ground for many a conspiracy theory, however, an already susceptible population with given fears, desires and a mechanistic world view were in need of such a rationale to support their existing state of mind. This was the time of the industrial revolution, we appeared to 'understand' machines, and phenomena in the natural world were going to be far easier to explain by making comparisons to our newfound technologies.

During the time of Pasteur a mechanical world was developing rapidly, with applications in almost every sphere of life, transport, consumer goods, farming, communication etc. People were beginning to explain their world by using machine-like analogies; the body itself was nothing more than a sophisticated machine. Blood transported by a pump - the heart, through the tubes and valves of the blood vessels, muscles acting on levers, nerve impulses acting like electric currents through the wiring of our nerves. We were a long way from understanding the interconnectedness of our systems and the effects of our emotions and mental facultles on the body. And as promoted by Descartes since the 17th century, consciousness itself was nothing more than a ghost within the mechanical body and for some people nothing more than an effect of the mechanical body itself.

By the time of Pasteur in the 1870's, all Western Europe was more or less industrialized, the coming of electricity and cheap steel after 1850 further speeded the process. According to Professor G Rempel of Western New England College, The Industrial Revolution may be defined as the application of power-driven machinery to manufacturing.

Between 1780 and 1860 many textile processes were mechanized. By 1812 the cost of making cotton yarn had dropped nine-tenths, and by 1800 the number of workers needed to turn wool into yarn had been reduced by four-fifths. And by 1840 the labor cost of making the best woolen cloth had fallen by at least half.

The steam engine provided a landmark in the industrial development of Europe. The first modern steam engine was built by an engineer Thomas Newcomen, in 1705, to improve the pumping equipment used to eliminate seepage in tin and copper mines. In 1763 James watt, an instrument-maker for Glasgow University, began to make improvements on Newcomen's engine. In 1774 the industrialist Michael Boulton took Watt into partnership, and their firm produced nearly five hundred engines before Watt's patent expired in 1800. Waterpower continued in use, but the factory was now liberated from the streamside where water mills had previously been the source of factory power.

The power of the steam engines were then harnessed in the development of steam trains and the coming of the railroads greatly facilitated the industrialization of Europe. After 1800 flat tracks were in use outside London, Sheffield, and Munich. With the expansion of commerce, facilities for the movement of goods from the factory to the ports or cities came into pressing demand. By 1830 a railway was opened from Liverpool to Manchester; and on this line George Stephenson's "Rocket" pulled a train of cars at fourteen miles an hour.

As early as 1831 Michael Faraday demonstrated how electricity could be mechanically produced, however through the nineteenth century the use of electric power was limited but the electrification of Europe proceeded apace in the twentieth century.

The ideas linking the function of microbes within the human body to nutrition, toxins, hormones and emotions were slightly more sophisticated than popular 19th century Western thinking. In many ways these notions sit far more comfortably within the realms of present day holistic thinking and the interconnected universe of modern physics. They were however too advanced for the machine-like analogies used to explain the workings of the human body in the 19th century. Béchamp was going to find it hard to translate his ideas to the man on the street; this may have contributed to the popularity of Pasteur's germ theory and the relative demise of Béchamp's soil theory.

However, there may be other considerations regarding human behaviour that would account for the popularity of Pasteur. There is, within us all, a powerful resistance to change, an inertia and momentum that makes it easier to keep on doing what we've been doing. This particular human phenomenon would seriously influence our choices, given the following options:

> A 'germ theory' approach would place the responsibility for the illness on an external agent of disease; the solution would lie in the extermination of the microbe, with no requirement to change anything on our part. Germ theory would give us the option to take no responsibility for our situation in our treatment of disease.

> Adopting a 'soil theory' of disease (where microbes create symptoms of disease according to the conditions within the body) would lead us to acknowledge the role of diet, nutrition, hormones, toxins, lifestyle, etc. As such, addressing the problem of disease would require change on our part.

For many individuals in both 19th century Europe and equally in today's society, we have to consider what would be the most attractive option, would it be the one that allows us to blame something else and take no responsibility for our state of 'disease'? As such, the disease would have nothing to do with 'us'; we could combat the disease by simply annihilating the germ. Consequently we could make disease a thing that exists outside of us, the result of something that had nothing to do with us, therefore requiring remedial action that did not involve 'us' having to do anything as drastic as 'change'. It was not through scientific enquiry, research and experimentation that lead us to embrace Pasteur and marginalize Béchamp, therefore… was it a result of this psychological desire for Pasteur to be right?

If, as promoted by Pasteur, infecting germs were primarily responsible for illness then the way to treat the illness would be to eradicate the germs (kill them by the use of toxic chemical agents) and avoid infection by avoiding contamination i.e. by avoiding contact with people that are infected. The disease becomes the microbe; they become synonymous with each other, to have measles is to have measles virus and to have the virus is to have the illness. Even though most people have viruses and bacteria and do not have the disease, because having the virus and to having the illness are in fact two separate issues. We can therefore talk about the possibility of giving someone the illness because in the Pasteur paradigm, the illness is no longer anything to do with our susceptibility or state of health, but some 'thing' that we can catch and transfer from one unsuspecting host to another.

We can be given an illness like an inanimate object, an item of clothing or a piece of machinery, equally the illness itself becomes externalised as some thing, no doubt, that if malfunctioning, could be left on the physician's desk to study and investigate. 'It' can be sorted out whilst the patient is able to deal with more important things and no doubt carry on doing the same things that created the illness in the first place, so that with the right drug the illness will be fixed. As such 'it' will have nothing to do with their life; undoubtedly somebody else would have given 'it' to them. This may seem the more attractive option, rather than blaming oneself, far easier to blame someone else, some irresponsible or unsuspecting individual responsible for spreading disease around the community.

If on the other hand, as demonstrated by Béchamp, the soil, i.e. our susceptibility, (the state of health of the individual) is primarily important for the contraction of an infectious disease, then treatment relies upon restoring balance and addressing the primary cause of this susceptibility. This would involve addressing issues of nutrition, sanitation (i.e. reduction of toxicity), mental and emotional wellbeing, physical rest, relaxation and other environmental factors. Therefore, according to the principles of Béchamp, you could never in fact contract anything that you were not already susceptible to and you could never resolve an illness simply by killing microbes. The illness would be inextricably linked to you.

At this point in history in the late 19th century there were no mass produced vaccinations, no antibiotics, no large pharmaceutical companies and therefore, on the face of it, no real scope for commercial conspiracy over and above the opposing commercial interests of the orthodox medical profession and the natural health, hygiene and food industries; yet, as a culture we invested in one approach far more than in the other. The approach was obviously that of Pasteur's.

Did we invest in this approach because of the available evidence of what actually worked or was it a calculated investment in an approach that if successful would reap many within the profession financial benefit and the governing authorities, power to deal with illness by simply handing out medication? Germ theory was not only an attractive option for individuals but also for governments, the 'success to effort' ratio appeared infinitely greater in the Pasteur paradigm than in Béchamp's.

In the Pasteur paradigm, where germs infect people and cause disease, governments were faced with the possibility of dealing with society's ills by simply investing in the production of the correct medication for the correct disease. This could then of course be administered en masse for a relatively small investment per individual; we would have the prospect of immediate reductions in disease, within the term of government. Government would have the possibility of success, without the tedium of having to deal with all those inconvenient, social and environmental issues of sanitation, food, shelter and social well-being. A germ theory of disease made the solutions to our troubles seem so much easier, and during the industrial revolution of 19th century Europe there were many social problems.

"They ruined us…They conquered continents.
We filled their uniforms… We cruised the seas.
We worked their mines…and made their histories.
You work, we rule, they said…We worked; they ruled.
They fooled the tenements…All men were fooled."

Douglas Dunn

The Industrial Revolution brought with it an increase in population and a shift from country to town dwelling. Between 1800 and 1950 most large European cities exhibited spectacular growth. At the beginning of the nineteenth century there were scarcely two dozen cities in Europe with a population of 100,000, but by 1900 there were more than 150 cities of this size.

The rapid growth of the cities brought some apparent advantages to the population but not without considerable cost to most people. The factory towns of England tended to become rookeries of jerry-built tenements, while the mining towns became long monotonous rows of company-built cottages, furnishing minimal shelter and little more.

The bad living conditions in the towns can be traced to lack of good brick, the absence of building codes, and the lack of machinery for public sanitation. But, it must be added, they were mainly due to the factory owners' tendency to regard laborers as commodities and not as a group of human beings.

Generally speaking, wages were low and hours were long, whilst working conditions were unpleasant and dangerous, with many businesses exploiting child-labour. For many, illnesses were a direct result of their living conditions; however, the wealthy factory owners owed their wealth to the exploitation of this new social class, their workers. Government usually favoured the factory owners; therefore reform and protective legislation was a long time coming and only after considerable public pressure in the form of coordinated unions and new socialist political opposition.

Eventually public health measures were developed, but in the 19th century the medical paradigm adopted by the government, was one wherein illnesses were caused by attacking microbes...

...governments were prepared to search for the magic bullet, but less prepared to improve the social conditions that directly lead to illness, especially if ultimately that was to be at the expense of their wealthy friends.

Commercial interests in the 19th century played a huge role in promoting the germ paradigm, and still do, with the concomitant search for commercially successful drugs in an attempt at the eradication of disease.

However, if Béchamp were correct, then diseases in our communities could only be dealt with by addressing those environmental issues: Workers hours would need to be cut, minimum ages introduced, pay increased, housing and sanitation improved, nutritious foods made readily available, and worse still, given the individual nature of susceptibility, therapeutic intervention would have to be tailor-made to each individual. All of which entailed far too much work and far too much investment from the government's wealthy friends for the uncertain prospect of the communities' future health.

> *"I do not know of any environmental group in any country that does not view its government as an adversary"*

> GH Brundtland 1989
> Three term Prime Minister of Norway (1981, 1986, 1990)
> International leader in sustainable development & public health.
> Served as the Director General of the World Health Organization

We as individuals wanted germ theory to be right, as governments and commercial business owners, we needed it to be right, we had our agenda... and our hero, Pasteur, was more than willing to champion the cause. An expert in self-publicity and adept at promoting what we wanted to hear, Pasteur, was clearly not the first to develop these ideas, nor the most knowledgeable; he was, however endorsing the right ideas, in the right places, at the right time, and more than willing to make financial profit from the whole endeavour.

> *"Let me tell you the secret that has led me to my goal. My strength lies solely in my tenacity"*
>
> Louis Pasteur

In March 1886 after enquiries into many deaths from his rabies vaccine Pasteur told Dr Navarre:

> *"From now on I won't accept discussion of my theories and my method. I won't have anyone coming to monitor my experiments".*
>
> Louis Pasteur

However the powers that be had decided, the theories of Pasteur were to be extolled and promoted, germs were the new public enemies and governments were to invest in techniques for their eradication.

So what exactly was being proposed when we decided to embark upon this journey of eradicating illness by killing microbes and the later development of vaccines?

CHAPTER THREE

3 How scientific is the theory of vaccines?

"A fact is a simple statement that everyone believes. It is innocent, unless found guilty. A hypothesis is a novel suggestion that no one wants to believe. It is guilty, until found effective."

Edward Teller

Hungarian-American theoretical physicist (1908-2003)
Jahn–Teller effect & BET theory, still mainstays in physics & chemistry.

3.1 The development of vaccines – "Guilty until proven effective"

The first mass smallpox vaccine campaign was introduced to the UK in 1840 and the subsequent mass vaccination policies have been generally recognized as being responsible for safely and effectively, reducing and eradicating diseases world-wide.

If we take a closer look at the history of vaccination we shall see that from the outset our vaccine legend appears to have been based on some historical manipulation, a manoeuvring designed to gloss over some inconvenient truths. The medical consensus would have us believe that the whole vaccination procedure was a technique first developed by Edward Jenner, and the inaugurating product was at once a glorious success.

3.1.1 Edward Jenner

During the era of Pasteur it was generally believed that individuals obtained immunity to certain illnesses, only after having contracted that particular illness; this would often confer life-long immunity. But although immunity and a reduced susceptibility to illness was a possible consequence of contracting an illness naturally, there also appeared to be associated risks. Risks that we are told are unknown, difficult to quantify and consequently difficult to influence in our favour. Edward Jenner lived throughout the scourge of smallpox, and in 1796 he was credited with having made the observation that the milkmaids with a history of cowpox infection, would not subsequently contract smallpox.

Cowpox was a mild skin disease believed to be contracted from skin contact with the microbes on the udders of cows, during the milking process, whereas smallpox was a dreaded disease manifesting unsightly pustules on the skin, was difficult to treat and with a high incidence of fatalities. The aftermath often affected the appearance of the skin, and could lead to chronic disorders and other adverse effects. Edward Jenner thought he had discovered the mechanism behind the porcelain beauty of milkmaids, having contracted cowpox they were then immune to smallpox and could never be defaced by this dreaded condition.

It was thought that the microbe responsible for cowpox was similar to the microbe responsible for smallpox. Therefore Jenner deduced that the human immune response to cowpox was also effective against smallpox. Having contracted cowpox an individual would be immune to future contact with smallpox; he therefore hypothesised that if he could get individuals to contract cowpox they would be protected against smallpox. On the face of it, a reasonable hypothesis and given the lack of clinical success at treating smallpox, it would appear to be a hypothesis well worth pursuing.

This would form the initial basis for the development of vaccination, however, it is worth noting at this point, that many doctors and members of the public rejected the idea of immunity to smallpox from natural cowpox, as they could testify to having cowpox and yet still contracted smallpox in later life.

Lily Loat writing extensively on the history of smallpox and vaccination states:

The great sanitarian Sir Edwin Chadwick maintained:

> "That cases of smallpox, of typhus, and of others of the ordinary epidemics, occur in the greatest proportion, in common conditions of foul air from stagnant putrefaction, from bad house drainage from sewers of deposit, from excrement-sodden sites, from filthy street surfaces, from impure water, and from overcrowding in private houses and in public institutions. That the entire removal of such conditions by complete sanitation and by improved dwellings is the effectual preventive of disease of these species, and of ordinary as well as extraordinary epidemic visitations" (From an address on "Prevention of Epidemics" delivered by Mr Chadwick at the Brighton Health Congress, 14th Dec. 1881.).

One of the most noted epidemiologists, Dr. August Hirsch, maintained that:

> "Smallpox, as well as typhus, takes up its abode most readily in those places where the noxious influences due to neglected hygiene make themselves most felt."

Loat further contends that:

> "The tradition of the dairymaids as to the protection afforded by cowpox against smallpox was rejected by many of Jenner's own medical acquaintances because they knew of numerous cases where those who had had cowpox subsequently developed smallpox."

But as far as Jenner was concerned, the principle remained an attractive possibility for disease prevention and he therefore carried out a number of experiments trying to develop a safe and effective method of extracting the pus or lymph from the skin eruption of individuals with cowpox and administering this to others in the hope of creating immunity to smallpox.

This injection of pus from cowpox vesicles into individuals as a form of preventative medication against smallpox has been credited as the first type of vaccination from this procedure and from the Latin, vaccinia = cow, we derive the term vaccination. The orthodox interpretation of medical history puts Jenner at the forefront of vaccine research, however a closer look at the historical evidence reveals otherwise; the practice of inoculating, by using the extract of a disease product to try and stimulate immunity in another patient was well known in Jenner's day. Jenner would have used various forms of inoculation in his own practise, in fact the specific cowpox version credited to Jenner was in fact used by Benjamin Jesty (1737-1816), of Yetminster in Dorset, and he was reputed to have performed successful cow-pox vaccination in 1774, thus preceding Jenner by more than twenty years.

The extent of the use of inoculations prior to Edward Jenner (1796) can be illustrated by looking at the "Lecture Memoranda,"XVII International Congress of Medicine, London, 1913, which states:

> "The practice of inoculation for the prevention of disease is one of considerable antiquity. The period of its discovery can only be conjectured..."

"Dhanwantari, the Vedic Father of Medicine, and the earliest known Hindu physician, who lived about 1,500 B.C., is supposed to have been the first to practice inoculation for smallpox. It is even stated that the ancient Hindus employed a vaccine, which they prepared by the transmission of the smallpox virus through a cow." (History of Inoculation and Vaccination, pp. 6, 13)

Dr. Clements in his pamphlet, "A Superstitious Custom" traces the inoculation practices through the various modern countries previous to Jenner's day (1796):

> Denmark in 1673 and later in 1778; Wales in 1722; France in 1712, and prohibited in 1763; Ireland in 1723; Germany in 1724; Italy in 1754 and 142 years later in 1896 (100 years after Jenner's smallpox vaccine).

Carlo Ruta, Professor of Materia Medica at the University of Perugia, Italy, protested against the deadly custom in these scathing words:

> "Vaccination is a monstrosity, a misbegotten offspring of error and ignorance; and, being such, it should have no place in either hygiene or medicine.... Believe not in vaccination, it is a world-wide delusion, an unscientific practice, a fatal superstition with consequences measured today by tears and sorrow without end."
>
> "In Ancient Greece and Rome, the MIGHTY NATIONS OF MIGHTY MEN, there was no inoculation — no vaccination — and no smallpox." These nations have been known down through history as being famous for their general habits of health, cleanliness and stability as well as their vigour and strength. Among the Greeks and Romans smallpox was unknown until it was carried there by the inoculators from other countries."

However in Baron's "Life of Jenner", (Vol. II, p. 304) we learn that:

> "On the 14th of May, 1796, Jenner vaccinated James Phipps, a boy about eight years old, with the matter taken from the hand of a dairymaid infected with casual cow-pox. The boy was thus vaccinated and this was to be tested at some point in the future by artificially infecting him with smallpox. (Note he was not to be tested by being exposed to the conditions of the natural disease or in times of epidemic but by injecting with smallpox pus). After waiting six weeks Jenner injected this boy on both arms with smallpox matter, (taken from the arm of a boy with smallpox) this was the first dose of artificial disease. Several months later Phipps was again injected with smallpox pus, he had, according to Jenner, been artificially exposed to the disease a second time and no effect was produced."

The artificial exposure to smallpox didn't result in symptoms of smallpox, so, on the strength of this one experiment and its questionable interpretation; Jenner based his claim that one vaccination would "forever secure a person from smallpox." No extensive time had elapsed to prove whether this was likely; but without this proof or any scientific basis or evidence for its practice, the doctors and the government adopted it and eventually made it compulsory, as Baron points out ..."no doubt, seeing the gold mine in profits that it would yield".

Convinced of the virtue of vaccination Edward Jenner inoculated his 18-month-old son with swinepox, on November 1791 and again in April 1798 with cowpox, he died of tuberculosis at the age of 21. James Phipps was declared immune to smallpox but he also died of tuberculosis at the age of 20.

Lilly Loat in her book "The Truth About Vaccination and Immunization" published in 1951...

"In every pro-vaccinist publication Jenner's great labours are extolled. There is no truth whatever in these tributes to his long study and experiment. Sir Benjamin Ward Richardson, although a believer in vaccination, well summed up the position as follows:

It is truly painful to say that the common opinion about the great labour of experiment, to which Jenner submitted himself, before he announced what is wrongly called his discovery, is mere childish adulation. His experiments are enumerated by himself, and may be put with observations without experiment, at 23; so that compared with the intense labour by which researches of a physiological kind are ordinarily carried out; they really rank as nothing in respect of labour (Disciples of Aesculapius-Jenner, 1900, pp 397-398).

However dubious the experiments and medical reasoning surrounding the use of vaccines, the 'Authorities' had decided, vaccines were to be the new wonder drugs. They heralded a new era of possibility with regard to preventative medicine; with the hope of producing further vaccines capable of eliminating illness and averting countless loss of life, counteracting the indiscriminate advance of infectious disease, and Jenner was to be the main publicist. Like Pasteur, his claim to fame lay in his ability to promote the practice of vaccination; his understanding of vaccines and disease prevention was however not his main forte, in practice he had many problems.

Administering cowpox microbes to an individual, in the form of a vaccine, was supposed to mimic the contraction of the natural disease 'cowpox', which would then create an immune response that would make the person immune to 'smallpox'. In order to produce such a vaccine Jenner had to collect sufficient cowpox microbes, he therefore decided to manufacture this vaccine by extracting the pus from the skin eruptions of individuals with cowpox; this pus was often referred to as 'lymph'.

However, distinguishing the exact nature of the disease from which this lymph could be extracted, was much more difficult than it appeared; there were in fact different types of pox illnesses in humans that were clinically very similar to cowpox i.e. although these illnesses involved different microbes they looked the same and produced the same symptoms. In addition, there were similar pox illnesses that could in fact be contracted from different animals. Vaccines had to be mass produced, it was not possible to wait around for volunteers to turn up with what appeared to be cowpox, extracting lymph on an individual and ad hoc basis. The pustular extraction (lymph) used in the production of smallpox vaccines needed to be standardised in order to replicate its therapeutic effects and since different illnesses in different animals would contain different microbes it was imperative to find out which pox illness was the one similar to smallpox in humans.

Jenner having changed his ideas on at least two occasions eventually insisted that the true protective variety was derived only from a disease known as "the grease "—the matter being transferred from the horse to the teats of the cow by men milkers after they had been attending to diseased horses.

An inquiry by the Lancet in the year 1900 into the "lymph" issued by thirteen establishments disclosed the fact that there was not one brand that was bacteriologically pure. In some there were hundreds of colonies of extraneous germs. The Lancet of May 13, 1922, wrote:

> Abroad, in place of the rabbit, the ass or the mule is employed, and the resulting ass-pox or mule-pox is used as the exalted seed stock for the vaccination of calves. Such lymph is freely admitted to the United Kingdom for the purpose of sale, and no practitioner knows whether the lymph he employs is derived from smallpox, rabbit-pox, ass-pox or mule-pox.

> Since Government lymph has been treated with glycerine, much of the official lymph must contain a certain amount of glycerine. What the remainder consists of no one can say. No microscopical examination can indicate which is the special germ (if there is one) of vaccine. One sample of lymph may be teeming with dangerous poisons; another may be almost innocuous and others contain no microbes at all. Dr. Kelsch, in a communication to the French Academy of Medicine (5 July 1909), told of his amazement to find typical vaccinal pustules on heifers inoculated with glycerine only.

> No attempt at standardisation of vaccine lymph has ever been made or could ever be made. How much impurity a sample has gathered up on its way from a human being through a calf or a donkey or a mule or a rabbit, perhaps then through a child and back to a calf again (or nowadays through a sheep), no one pretends to know. No vaccinator can state with certainty the composition of a tube of "pure glycerinated lymph." He is experimenting with a mixture that may be so dangerous as to cause death, but he knows nothing about it. The Therapeutic Substances Regulations make no attempt to define vaccine lymph. They say, in effect, that vaccine lymph is "vaccine lymph."

The results of Jenner's experiments were debated at length; clearly there were serious inadequacies in the production and standardisation of the vaccine, in addition there were few conclusive experiments able to satisfy the most basic scientific enquiry. However, the government, seemingly very attached to the possibility of this miracle form of protection, pushed forward with the production of the vaccine and the eventual passing of legislation making smallpox vaccination a legal requirement for all UK citizens. From 1867 evaders of vaccination were to be prosecuted.

3.1.2 'Vaccination' enters the Encyclopaedia Britannica

The overwhelming consensus is that smallpox vaccination was a great success, representing a significant milestone in medicines triumph over illness, eventually eradicating smallpox from the entire world. In fact the success of smallpox vaccination is so enshrined in medical history that most doctors and scientists are very rarely concerned enough to investigate the matter further.

One such doctor Dr Creighton was commissioned by the Editors of the *Encyclopaedia Britannica* to write an article on vaccination for the ninth edition. (In 1889 he also published his views in a more popular form in a work entitled *Jenner and Vaccination:* Cassell & Co.), In a letter to the press in 1895 he states:

> *"Having written medical articles in The Encyclopaedia Britannica regularly from the year 1880, I was engaged in the ordinary course to write on vaccination, ... I had hardly begun work upon vaccination in 1886 when I found myself immersed in an original inquiry into the nature and circumstances of the historical cowpox of Jenner and others.*

The information available to Dr Creighton was so ambiguous that he had to research the original data himself, leading to an extensive review of the available scientific literature. He goes on to say...

... One result of the historical and pathological research was that I began to suspect the value of cowpox as a protective from smallpox... The article was sent in soon after, and was in due course put into type.

Unfortunately for pro-vaccinators Dr Creighton could make no excuse for what he concluded was <u>the failure of vaccination</u>. Dr. Creighton also informed the Royal Commission (Q5584) that up to 1886, when the article on vaccination in the Encyclopaedia Britannica was written, he had no doubt about the value of vaccination, that it never occurred to him to question the thing at all, and that he took it as one of the things he had been taught as a student. He left the Commission in no doubt as to the result of his studies.

"In my opinion," he said (Q-5430) "vaccination affords no protection against smallpox."

Dr Creighton an eminent doctor who had written countless articles for the Encyclopaedia Britannica, had wholeheartedly believed in the value of vaccines, had been taught the virtue of vaccinations in medical school, practised medicine for many years and had seen no reason to doubt their safety and efficacy. Now, only after conducting his own research, discovered that they were effectively useless.

Dr. Creighton died on the 18th July 1927, 80 years old. The following brief extracts from an obituary notice appeared in the *Lancet* on the 30th July, 1927, written by Prof. William Bulloch, F.R.S: —

"By the death of Charles Creighton, England has lost her most learned medical scholar of the nineteenth century, although it cannot be forgotten that some of his opinions were the subject of such criticism that he ceased to be felt as a power in the medical world . . .. I was his only intimate friend for years before he died, for he was a most lonely forsaken man. To the end he was a scholar and a philosopher and the most learned man I ever knew. He spoke and read nearly all the European languages and had an extraordinary knowledge not only of medicine but of the classics and the Bible. His knowledge of English literature and history was also profound. Although he frequently spoke as if he wished to be considered and remembered as a pathologist, it is by his History of Epidemics in Great Britain that he earned a permanent place beside the great masters of medical history like Daremberg, Haeser, Freind, and Hirsch. In my judgment Creighton's History of Epidemics is the greatest work of medical learning published in the nineteenth century by an Englishman.

"The real tragedy of Creighton's life was connected with his views on cowpox and vaccination...His article on 'Vaccination' in the ninth edition of the Encyclopedia Britannica, published in 1888, literally sealed Creighton's fate. Based on an extended study of the original data, he came to the conclusion that Jenner's work was incorrect, and that cowpox was not, as Jenner stated, 'Variola Vaccine (not related to smallpox).' In Creighton's view cowpox had nothing to do with smallpox and was not a protective against smallpox.

"The issue between Creighton and general professional opinion on vaccination was not thrashed out there and then as it ought to have been. It was deemed more expedient to drop Creighton into oblivion, and if he was ever referred to at all it was only as 'Creighton the Anti-Vaccinator.' All his other work was forgotten in the debacle, and he was a doomed man...in the opinion of many he was harshly treated by the world for holding views that did not conform to standard. Perhaps this very world has become more tolerant than it was in Creighton's time, because even in his own subject there are epidemiologists who express with impunity to-day views as heterodox as those for which Creighton was pilloried and ostracised 40 years ago."

In spite of, rather than because of, the evidence government health policy makers came to the conclusion that smallpox vaccination was an effective public health procedure and in principle the ideas of Jenner have remained with us to the present day. This does lead us to question the source of this apparent medical prejudice; why did governments persist in such an apparently flawed medical policy? And more significantly, are we today, over 150 years later, still locked in an old paradigm promoting heath policies that have long since proven to be ineffective or have we learnt from our mistakes? Have more recent developments in medical research made up for our previous inadequacies?

3.1.3 Discovering the antibody

Subsequent to these observations, research in both Germany and Japan (1890) resulted in the discovery of the 'antibody', an immune protein that could be produced by certain immune cells called B cells. They were apparently produced in response to specific foreign microbes that had entered the blood. These antibodies were able to physically wrap around certain portions of the infecting microbe producing a kind of mirror image copy, they would fit the invading microbe very much like a lock and key.

As preparation for future invasions by these microbes, great numbers of identical copies of these antibodies would then be reproduced. They would remain in the blood and would have the ability to recognise future microbes of the same type. These antibodies were then thought to be responsible for the destruction and elimination of the invading microbe. Should there be any subsequent invasion of these microbes then the human body, with the help of these pre-formed antibodies, would be able to destroy and eliminate them easily without the need for fully developed symptoms.

This <u>antibody memory</u> was considered to be a major breakthrough in the understanding of the immune response and was thought to be the method by which future infections could be dealt with more easily than the first. Hence people were thought to be immune once they had developed antibodies to specific foreign elements; toxins or microbes. This discovery was deemed to be so significant that it was further deduced you could only be immune to something your immune system had previously been in contact with and therefore had antibodies to.

Unlike the original vaccine against smallpox, in which cowpox microbes were used because they were thought to be similar to smallpox microbes, the vaccines that we manufacture against the later illnesses were not created from similar microbes, but generally taken from a culture (a growth) of the same microbe or toxin thought to be responsible for the disease. Some vaccines are made from bacteria, for example whooping cough, some by viruses e.g. measles and others by the toxins of bacteria e.g. tetanus. For the purposes of discussing vaccines in general we shall call all of these different viruses, bacteria and toxins, 'pathogens', agents associated with disease.

So, if we were creating a measles vaccine, rather than trying to find a similar supposedly less virulent virus from another illness, as we tried to do with cowpox for the smallpox vaccine, we would try to create a culture of the actual measles virus. Because we use the real virus, we therefore have to deactivate it in some way, to avoid creating symptoms of disease when we inject it into the individual in the form of a vaccine. This process of deactivation depends on the type of pathogen being used, bacteria, virus or toxin and would involve heat, mechanical or chemical deactivation.

This deactivated pathogen is then injected (except for some oral vaccines) into our blood, in the hope that we would produce antibodies that are similar enough to the antibodies that would be created to the real pathogen. These antibodies would hopefully recognise subsequent infections of the real thing and therefore protect us from fully developing symptoms of the actual disease.

The conventional interpretation of the developments and conclusions arrived at so far will therefore illustrate the standard medical context from which most of us understand health, immunity and infectious illness today.

> The germ (microbe) is primarily responsible for infectious illness and can be transferred from one person to another. Therefore illness itself can be transferred from one person to another.
> Different microbes cause their own specific illness and therefore infectious illnesses are classified according to the type of microbe.
> Some microbes are more dangerous than others and can cause serious illnesses, even in healthy individuals.
> The formation of antibodies to microbes is indicative of an effective immune response; therefore one important goal in the prevention of illness is to stimulate the production of antibodies.

From the above it was further deduced that:

> The detection and measurement of antibody levels in an individual gives a measure of immunity within that individual.
> Immunity to an illness cannot be gained unless you have been exposed to the microbe and therefore produced antibodies to it.

These notions seem perfectly feasible given the progress made so far. However, more recent developments in our understanding of health and illness significantly alter these fundamental premises.

3.1.4 Vaccine Production

When administering any chemical substance into the human body, because of the infinitely complex nature of chemical interactions, there will always be unforeseen and unwanted physiological effects known as 'side effects'. However, regardless of side effects, in the production of vaccines, we are faced with an inherent dilemma.

In order to produce a safe vaccine from a particular pathogen, (virus, bacteria or toxin), we have to deactivate the pathogen in a way that reduces its ability to produce symptoms of the disease. We want the body to recognise it as the real thing and produce antibodies, but we don't want it to be capable of doing any damage, hence the dilemma:

➢ If the pathogen is not changed enough i.e. not deactivated enough, then we risk injecting problematic agents into our bodies which would produce the symptoms of illness, the very thing we are trying to avoid. Perhaps producing even more severe consequences due to the nature of cultivating the pathogen and presenting this to the body in an unnatural way, via an injection.

➢ However, if, during the deactivation process in the production of the vaccine, we change the pathogen too much, then the antibodies we produce in our bodies in response to these elements will be a mirror image of a vastly different pathogen. Therefore, should we come in contact with the real pathogen at some point in the future, the antibodies will not recognise them and according to our immune theory we would not have immunity.

It is therefore imperative that we test both the safety and effectiveness of each specific vaccine, given the possible outcomes as described above.

3.1.5 Effectiveness of vaccines

Initially, efficacy studies carried out on vaccines are 'in vitro' studies (i.e. trials carried out in laboratory test tubes). They are designed to find out whether the pathogen that is cultured and changed in the production of a vaccine actually stimulates antibody production, then, whether these antibodies are capable of recognising and attaching to the real pathogen.

Once the results to these initial experiments are positive we assume that we have a potentially viable vaccine. That is we have a vaccine that is capable of stimulating certain cells of the body to produce antibodies that will attach to what we believe is the cause of the disease. Vaccine producers will then go on to test these vaccines in real people, trying to assess if individuals are stimulated into producing viable antibodies (immunogenicity studies).

Of course, this does not tell us what happens to a real person over an extended period of time or in a real disease situation. We may produce antibodies to a potential pathogen but the real test is in whether we are less likely to contract the illness, will it be less severe if we do and are we necessarily healthier if we do not have the illness.

Unfortunately most of the studies and statistics quoted regarding the effectiveness of vaccines are obtained from these immunogenicity trials and test-tube (in vitro) studies. We have to be clear that such studies tell us very little about real people in real disease situations. Logically, in order draw worthwhile conclusions; a vaccine needs to undergo further trials evaluating safety and efficacy in real populations assessing the prevalence and severity of actual disease as opposed to numbers of antibodies to a pre-supposed pathogen.

3.1.6 Are antibodies necessary for immunity?

Further importance is added to the necessity of population studies in assessing vaccine safety and effectiveness when we consider the following:

> ➢ Antibodies in fact, form only a very small part of our total immune response. It is conceivable that individuals can respond successfully to germs and develop long-term immunity and yet have produced no detectable levels of antibody. Similarly it is conceivable that individuals that have produced high levels of antibodies may still not have successfully

developed immunity and may still contract the disease in the future.

This appears to be in direct contradiction to assumptions made so far and perhaps, one would think, not an opinion shared by the current medical establishment. However many people are surprised to learn that this is in fact standard medical text. For example, in correspondence with Dr Clements, Director of the World Health Organisation, Extended Program of Immunisations, in October 1995, I asked him to comment on the fact that an individual can have high levels of antibody and may not be immune, whilst others with no detectable levels can be immune. Dr Clements agreed and I quote…

"You are right to say there is not a precise relationship between seroresponse (production of antibodies) and protection… immunity can be demonstrated in individuals with very low or no detectable levels of antibody."

Dr Clements is still the current director of the WHO Extended Program of Immunisation.

Contrary to popular opinion it is not possible to use a test somebody's antibody levels to ascertain their level of immunity. Therefore it is likely that antibody production is not the best indicator of immunity and therefore there must be other equally, if not more, important factors involved in the immune response.

3.1.7 Vaccine safety

Initial safety trials on volunteers are carried out within fairly limited criteria. In the first instance, when assessing the safety of a vaccine, the adverse reactions researchers are looking for are, of course, going to be those similar to the symptoms of the disease being vaccinated against, there is a certain blinkered approach to the possibility of other adverse effects. For example when assessing the safety of a measles vaccine, researchers are more inclined to be looking for symptoms of measles with its known complications rather than the possibility of other symptoms.

Once the vaccine is in the population there are then acknowledged difficulties in assessing the incidence of adverse events by the relevant health authorities, this is mainly due to the reliance on 'voluntary' reports of adverse events sent in to the health authorities by doctors. It is interesting to note that in countries where reporting is compulsory, such as in France, the number of adverse events are higher than in countries like the UK, where reporting is voluntary.

However, the under-reporting of drug side-effects is a world-wide phenomenon, in 2006 the Drug research unit at Southampton University published a survey of reporting incidence in the international journal of toxicology and drug experience.

> In total, 37 studies using a wide variety of surveillance methods were identified from 12 countries. These generated 43 numerical estimates of under-reporting. The median under-reporting rate across the 37 studies was 94%.

> L.Hazell & S.A Shakir, (Drug safety 2006 29(5): 385-96)

A massive 94% of side-effects are consistently not reported around the world and the research team found that many of these are severe reactions to drugs.

The withdrawal of the Urabe strain of mumps virus used in MMR vaccine illustrates quite clearly the phenomena of under-reporting with regard to adverse effects. The Urabe strain used in the mumps component of the MMR vaccine was implicated in some cases of meningitis because the vaccine virus particles were isolated from the cerebrospinal fluid of affected children. Canada stopped using the vaccine in 1989. In the UK however, where alternative strains of mumps vaccine were not so readily available, the health authority wanted to study the situation before considering the withdrawal of the vaccine whilst they had nothing to replace it, therefore various studies were conducted to assess the risk.

Studies based on voluntary reports gave reassuringly low estimates, 1 case of mumps meningitis per 143,000 (notification by doctors) to 1 case in 250,000 (voluntary reports by paediatricians). So although there were cases of mumps meningitis being caused by the vaccine they were, according to the health authority, acceptably low. But when greater efforts were made to identify cases, for instance by cross-linking laboratory and hospital reports to vaccination records, the risk rose to between 1 in 4,000 (notification by doctors) and 1 in 21,000 (voluntary reports by paediatricians). These studies were reported by the UK Parliamentary office of science and technology and suggested significant under-reporting of vaccine-associated meningitis, which led to the withdrawal of the vaccine in 1992.

For many years MMR was therefore causing mumps meningitis in children and was essentially going unnoticed; its incidence was being under reported in some settings by a factor of 30. Thirty times more cases were found, using different methods of assessing the numbers of cases, and it took the withdrawal of the vaccine from another country before we noticed the problem in the UK. The main method used to assess the numbers of adverse events from vaccines, was through the use of voluntary reports made by doctors to the health authorities, essentially, doctors have to make the connection between a symptom and the vaccine and secondly admit to the connection between the health problem and the vaccine and finally to report it, all of which lead to significant under-reporting of that particular vaccine problem.

Perhaps researchers can be forgiven for not noticing and therefore not reporting the adverse effects of vaccines on individuals, especially if those effects appear to be unrelated to the illnesses being vaccinated against. The previous example of meningitis, is not a classical symptom of mumps and therefore not likely to be associated with the use of the mumps vaccine. Another example of this being, Lupus erythematosus, an autoimmune disease of the connective tissue, which has now been found to be associated with the Hepatitis B vaccine. Lupus is a self-destructive inflammatory condition with the formation of scar tissue often affecting the skin, heart, lungs and brain, whereas hepatitis is a condition affecting the liver.

However the USA National Academy of Sciences report into the side effects of vaccines published in September 1993 demonstrates that even when the adverse effects of the vaccine look similar to the symptoms of the vaccine illness, they are still being overlooked by the medical community.

The above 1993 report was written by an expert panel convened by the Academy's Institute of Medicine and was headed by Richard Johnston, a Yale University Paediatrician who stated that the "biggest surprise" was the evidence showing that tetanus and oral polio vaccine caused Guillain-Barré syndrome. However Guillain-Barré syndrome involves symptoms of paralysis and could in fact easily be mistaken for polio.

Which in itself, bears testimony to the negligence of the researchers into the safety of the vaccine and the surveillance system set up to monitor the adverse effects of vaccines. Polio and tetanus, although different illnesses are both characterised by symptoms of paralysis, Guillain-Barré also involves symptoms of paralysis. When vaccines are introduced into the population, at the very least, researchers would be looking at the incidence of symptoms that are similar to the symptoms of the illness being vaccinated against. Polio vaccine and tetanus vaccines were introduced, they were creating syndromes of paralysis (Guillain-Barré syndrome) and 30 - 40 years after the widespread introduction of these vaccines, in 1993, evidence of them causing paralysis was a "big surprise".

This, of course, is evidence of an extremely poor monitoring system and, as reported in New Scientist 25 September 1993, Joanne Hatem, who heads the USA Health Research Council in her comments of the above states: "The subtext of the report is that the FDA and CDC (the agencies involved in monitoring disease and drug reactions) have done a dismal job in following up and analysing reported reactions". So, not only are the reporting systems deficient but the analysis and follow up of those reported cases are also inadequate.

In the UK there has been much controversy over the findings of Dr Andrew Wakefield linking the use of MMR vaccine with regressive autism, a potentially severe and debilitating, behavioural and emotional condition. Consequently confidence in the vaccine has diminished considerably among the general public and the government health authorities have been at pains to try and restore faith in the vaccine. In 2001 the UK health authority publicised a report of a study conducted in Finland, citing this as proof that the MMR vaccine does not cause autism. However, closer examination of this study only serves to illustrate the problems associated with the governments prejudice and tunnel vision when assessing adverse effects of vaccines. The report appeared convincing, involving 1.8 million children over a 14-year period finding no link between MMR vaccine and autism. There were however major limitations to the study:

> Firstly the study relied on voluntary notifications of adverse effects, in which experts agree, at best; pick up 10% of incidents.
> Secondly the reactions that were being looked for; fits, allergies, neurological disorders, rheumatoid arthritis and diabetes – did not include autism or any symptoms associated with it.
> Thirdly the reported adverse reactions concentrated on a three-week period after vaccination and would therefore miss the slow appearance of symptoms associated with regressive autism.

The study was therefore completely inadequate in its ability to assess the incidence of regressive autism.

This Finnish report was not based on a study of the effects of MMR, it was not an independent research project on the effects of MMR on the human physiology, but a look at the reports sent in to the local health authorities. Reports that were <u>not</u> looking for autism or any symptoms associated with autism, in a time-frame outside of the normal appearance of symptoms, therefore highly unlikely to find any symptoms of autism associated with the use of MMR vaccine.

Yet the government cited this as scientific evidence that MMR does not cause autism. If we then take into account the fact that the report was supported by a grant from Merck & Co, USA, a producer of MMR vaccine we see that there have been inherent conflict of interest issues and that this was not an independent study. Furthermore the subsequent documents, aimed at restoring public confidence in MMR, distributed to doctors in the UK was authored by Mike Watson medical director of Aventis Pasteur also a manufacturer of MMR vaccine. This is of course worse than inadequate and appears to indicate a level of intentional neglect amounting to deceit.

Dr Michelle Odent working at the Primal Health Research Centre in London found a link between whooping cough vaccine and asthma; a report of which was published in The Journal of the American Medical Association in 1994. What astounded Dr Odent was the refusal of health authorities and other researchers to look into the effects of whooping cough vaccine in relation to the increase in asthma. In a public debate in London in which I was also a panel member, he expressed frustration at the authorities in looking at every other issue, dust, pollution, home furnishings…"even the colour of the carpet" but in no way are they willing to look at the possibility of vaccine damage.

Paul Shattock, OBE, Honorary Director of the Autism research Unit, at Sunderland University is similarly critical. In his research, he estimates that approximately 10% of autism in the UK is caused by the MMR vaccine, but he states that he is not allowed to research those cases that are due to the vaccine and the University will not publicly endorse those findings, even though they are willing to stand by his findings in other areas of research regarding autism.

Carol Stott, Department of Psychiatry, Cambridge University studied a cohort of children believed to be damaged by the MMR vaccine and found a significant link between the onset of autistic symptoms and the administration of MMR vaccine. The heads of the department at Cambridge University were similarly convinced of the link, suggesting, as Carol Stott did, that it required further study. However because GlaxoSmithKline (a manufacturer of MMR vaccine) funds research for Cambridge University Psychiatry department, Carol was told further research in that area would be like ..."sawing off the branch that holds us up." Carol Stott had to abandon the research.

This blinkered approach to the assessment of problems associated with vaccination would have been greater during the early days of vaccines, at a time when most of our safety data was obtained, and our knowledge of adverse events was even more limited. In fact most of the studies conducted on the vaccines used in the UK and other developed countries have come from under-developed parts of the world i.e. 'developing countries', the inadequacy of reporting has been illustrated by R.G.Hendrickse in The Transactions of The Royal Society of Tropical Medicine, as late as 1975 it is stated "No figures of vaccine risk are available from developing countries", this is not to be confused with no risk, but that no figures of risk are available. Which is an admission of a widespread and complete absence of adverse event monitoring, possibly something that no other pharmaceutical product could get away with. Vaccine manufacturers themselves admit to a level of adverse events occurring from all vaccines; over a number of years of vaccination, side effects were clearly being ignored or at least not connected to the use of vaccines.

In addition to this there are even more restrictions placed on the reporting of adverse events once the vaccine is in general use. Most health authorities with regard to vaccine compensation have agreed extremely short time limits, after which time adverse effects cannot be attributed to the vaccine. For live vaccines, adverse effects have to be noted within 14 days and for killed vaccines within 72 hours, any adverse event noted outside of this time would not be attributable to the vaccine. We know of many examples of reactions to medical intervention, drugs and toxins that take many months to fully develop within an individual, how can we possibly justify the use of these artificial time restraints?

Viera Scheibner, now a retired principal research scientist with a doctorate in Natural Sciences, is the author of the book 'Vaccination - The Medical Assault on the Immune System'. Her research shows quite clearly the problems associated with these artificial cut off points. Interested in researching and therefore preventing the incidence of sudden infant death syndrome (SIDS) Leif Carlson developed the cot-watch monitor, an instrument that was able to record the breathing patterns of babies whilst asleep, it could also sound an alarm if the pattern indicated undue stress in the child.

Viera Scheibner and Leif Carlson studied the results of these breathing traces and noticed that from the time of trauma, a consistent pattern of stressed breathing would occur, not only at the time of stress but also at periodic intervals afterwards, typically 2-3 days, 1 week and 3 weeks. Many experts working in this field are able to indicate the most likely day of trauma in a child, by studying the recordings of their sleep breathing patterns. Their predictions can be corroborated by the incidence of illness and death at those intervals after trauma.

To her surprise Viera Scheibner found that the day of trauma often coincided with the day of vaccination, when presenting these patterns to other researchers they would also confirm the day of trauma and were similarly shocked to learn that these would often coincide with the day of vaccination. However Viera experienced first hand the reluctance of doctors and other scientists to investigate this further, with many wanting to distance themselves from the implications this may have on vaccine policy. However this led Viera Scheibner to research the whole issue of vaccinations in much greater depth, and years of research culminated in the publication of her book, showing clearly a consistent pattern and the delayed nature of some of the effects of vaccines beyond the time limits set by health authorities.

The subject of 'cot death' is a phenomenon that we are told remains a complete medical mystery:

> *Cot death (sudden infant death syndrome, SIDS) = the sudden unexpected death of an infant less than two years old (peak occurrence between two and six months) from an unidentifiable cause. (Oxford Medical Dictionary)*

Investigations of Viera Scheibner uncovered some interesting facts:

> *Between 1970 and 1974, 37 infant deaths occurred after DPT vaccination in Japan; because of this the doctors in one prefecture boycotted vaccination (Iwasa et al. 1985 and Noble et al. 1987). Consequently, the Japanese Government first stopped DPT vaccination for 2 months in 1975, and, when vaccination was resumed, the vaccination age was lifted to 2 years.*

> *Interestingly, not only the entity of sudden death virtually disappeared from vaccine injury compensation claims (only 2 deaths were the subject of vaccine injury compensation claims in the 2-year olds compared with 37 in younger children), but the overall infant mortality has improved:*

> *Japan zoomed from 17th to first place in infant mortality in the world. This means that Japan moved from a very high bracket to the lowest infant mortality rate in the world (Jenny Scott 1991). Interestingly, Noble et al. (1987) who spent some 2 weeks in Japan studying the acellular whooping vaccine there, wrote that "It is difficult to exclude pertussis vaccines as a causal factor (in sudden infant death) even when other aetiologies are suggested, particularly when the adverse events occur in close temporal association with vaccination".*

Cot death, an event so devastating, a syndrome of which we have virtually no knowledge, and admittedly no definitive proof of a link to vaccine, however, rather than reserve judgement and investigate possible links to vaccines, health authorities feel confident to say that there is no link to vaccines and in spite of the knowledge that cot death and overall infant mortality declined in a country that at one point did not vaccinate below the age of two years.

Dr. Barthelow Classen, working in Finland found that diabetic problems occurred in statistically significant clusters three to four years after vaccines were administered. The more vaccines you are exposed to, the greater the risk of diabetes. "I am very confident that we have proven that vaccines are causing diabetes. We have tons of data now to support this, including randomized, controlled clinical trials."

There is a great deal of evidence showing the delayed nature of many of the problems associated with vaccines. To place very restricted and arbitrary deadlines on the time limit after which problems cannot be attributed to the vaccine will reduce the amount of reported problems, but will of course underestimate the real risks associated with vaccines. To know the risks we need proof and for that we require suitably designed long-term studies, following up patients for years and into the next generations.

In reporting these incidents Mark Sircus Ac., O.M.D. (Director of The International Medical Veritus Association) is similarly critical of this approach and says, "If children do not die or get chronically ill within three days (of vaccination) the present medical authorities feel confident and secure in telling the world multiple vaccines are safe."

We can conclude that in order to ascertain the effectiveness of vaccines, it is not adequate to rely on evidence relating to the production of antibodies. With regard to safety it is imperative to study the effects of vaccination for longer than the current time limits allow, whilst carefully looking at effects on the whole body. However in developing our story further we need to acknowledge the fact that vaccine promoters often quote declines in disease in various populations around the world as evidence of the effectiveness of vaccines...evidence from 'disease statistics'.

CHAPTER FOUR

4 What's wrong with the evidence for the success of vaccines?

> *"Do not put your faith in what statistics say, until you have carefully considered what they do not say."*
>
> William W. Watt

4.1 Disease statistics

There is a consensus among most people, both of the general public and medical professionals, that vaccines have been responsible for the decline in both the incidence of infectious diseases and in the severity of these illnesses (often indicated by the number of deaths - mortality). When looking at the efficacy of vaccines it is in fact rare that figures of antibody levels are quoted, the proof is in the pudding so to speak, in what actually happens to disease levels. The book "Immunisation against infectious disease" published by the UK Departments of Health (HMSO) has for many years presented graphs showing the incidence of several diseases and the apparent effects that the introduction of vaccines have had on these illnesses. For example the following graph shows that the incidence of diphtheria dropping since the introduction of the diphtheria vaccine in the 1940's:

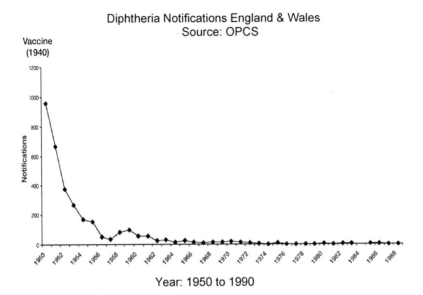

Diphtheria Notifications England & Wales
Source: OPCS

Vaccine
(1940)

Year: 1950 to 1990

However, to make a more worthwhile assessment we need to get a picture of what happened before the introduction of vaccines so that we may be able to see any discernable trends. Government sources say that they do not have reliable figures of incidence from before the periods shown therefore are unable to present the bigger picture. Therefore the bigger picture is simply not presented.

There are, however, figures published regarding death rates of many of the illnesses, therefore by looking at mortality we can get a picture of the severity of those illnesses before and after vaccines. Using these figures that are obtained from the <u>same</u> office that supply the figures for the HMSO incidence graphs, we are able to show trends over a 100-year period as compared to a 20-year period. We can then see what effect vaccines have had on mortality and therefore severity of illnesses. (By looking later at the tuberculosis graph we can also see that severity and incidence do in fact follow parallel trends).

The following graph shows the decline in incidence in death rate of diphtheria before and after the introduction of diphtheria vaccine.

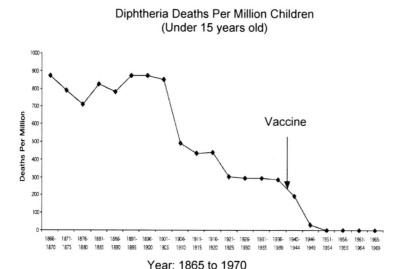

Diphtheria Deaths Per Million Children
(Under 15 years old)

Year: 1865 to 1970

For diphtheria at least, results showing a before and after trend, do not put the vaccine in such a favourable light. It is possible of course that the vaccine has had some effect, however, that now needs to be measured against a backdrop of what would have happened anyway. If we look at other illnesses presented in this manner we are able to demonstrate a similar effect.

Graph showing the incidence of whooping cough <u>from 1950</u> printed in "Immunisation against infectious disease" published by the UK Departments of Health (HMSO).

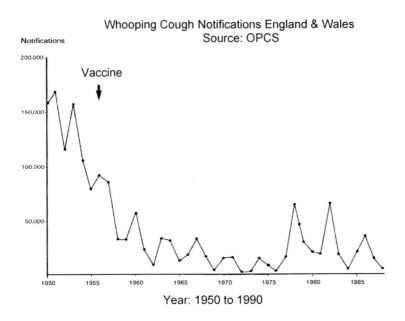

Year: 1950 to 1990

Graph showing death rate of whooping cough from 1850:

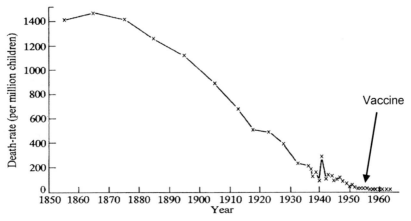

FIGURE 8.12. Whooping cough: death rates of children under 15: England and Wales.

Graph showing the incidence of tetanus <u>from 1970</u> printed in "Immunisation against infectious disease" published by the UK Departments of Health (HMSO).

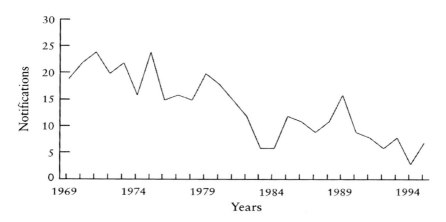

Tetanus notification to ONS
England and Wales (1969-1995)

Graph showing death rate of tetanus from 1905:

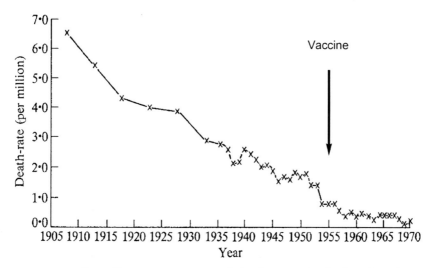

FIGURE 8.11. Tetanus: mean annual death rates: England and Wales.

Graph showing the incidence and death rates of tuberculosis <u>from 1940</u> printed in "Immunisation against infectious disease" published by the UK Departments of Health (HMSO).

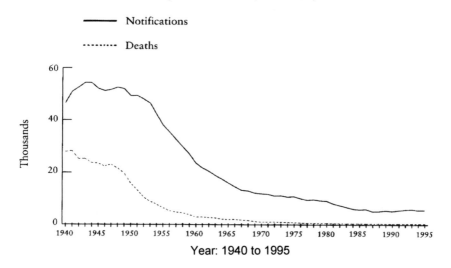

Notifications of tuberculosis and deaths to ONS
England and Wales (1940-1995)

——— Notifications

········ Deaths

Year: 1940 to 1995

Graph showing death rate of tuberculosis from 1838:

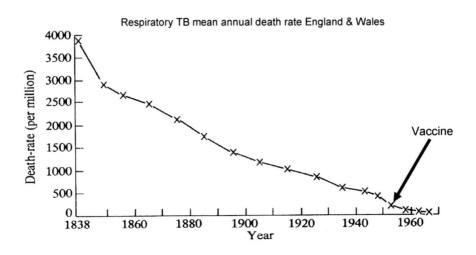

Respiratory TB mean annual death rate England & Wales

Vaccine

Graph showing the incidence of measles <u>from 1940</u> printed in "Immunisation against infectious disease" published by the UK Departments of Health (HMSO).

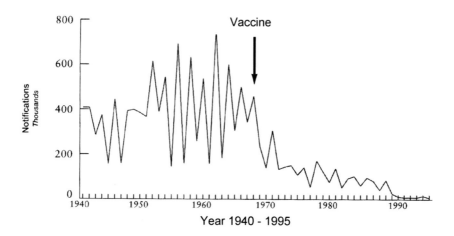

Graph showing death rate of measles from 1850:

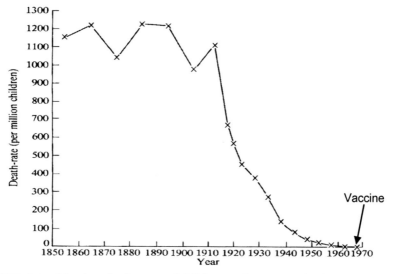

FIGURE 8.14. Measles: death rates of children under 15: England and Wales.

We can clearly see that in most instances, decline in severity (as indicated by death rate) was well over 95% BEFORE vaccines were ever introduced. It is also worth reiterating that these figures are from the same government departments that collate the incidence figures for the HMSO book quoted above. They are not separate studies conducted by different groups with different prejudices. Please also note that the figures relate to 'rates' i.e. deaths per specific number of population and are therefore automatically adjusted for population rises.

It is even more interesting to note that scarlet fever, the illness responsible for the largest number of childhood deaths in the early 19th century declined in severity to the extent that no deaths and negligible incidence occurred in the 1960's, there has **never been a vaccine developed for scarlet fever** and there has never been a return to high incidence or deaths.

Scarlet Fever Deaths Per Million Children (Under 15 Years Old)

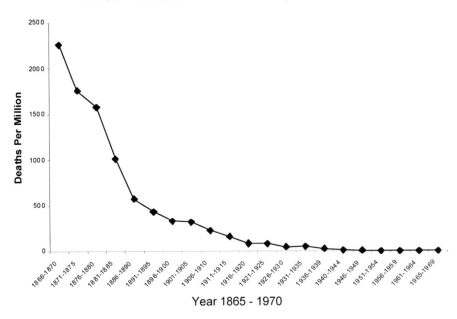

Year 1865 - 1970

It is very clear from the above that there are obviously other factors involved in the decline in severity <u>and</u> incidence of diseases, therefore if we are to introduce a medical procedure to a whole population, it is important to measure its effects against a backdrop of what would have happened anyway. Vaccine supporters claim to be scientific, wanting the most rigorous tests to prove that a vaccine could cause any harm yet seem to be very willing to accept flimsy data to suggest vaccine safety and efficacy.

We are often 'sold' medical procedures as though they are the only factors capable of dealing with illness, as though we have no natural immunity, and no natural tendency to heal.

This can sometimes take the form of statistical manipulation and scare mongering. On the 9th of January 2002, the following graph was printed in the Guardian as part of an article written by Sarah Boseley, The Guardian's Health Editor, telling us that <u>without vaccinating</u>…"measles, left to itself, tends to be cyclical – it would cause more than 100 deaths."

How vaccinations have reduced death

England and Wales

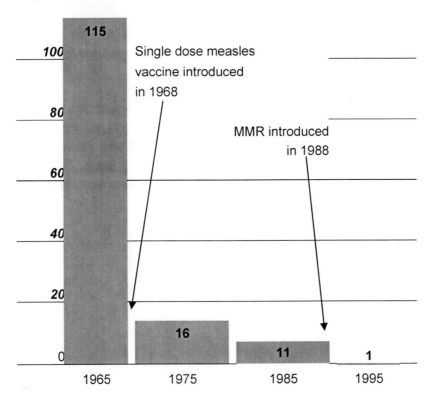

Source ONS

These figures refer to the UK and have been obtained from ONS the Office of National Statistics, previously called OPCS (Office of Population and Census Statistics), where in fact the previous graphs are taken from. We can see that the nature of the Guardian graph in omitting the trends before the vaccine, gives the impression that the decline was entirely due to the vaccine, lets look once more at the wider picture:

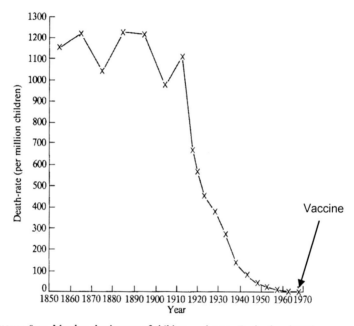

FIGURE 8.14. Measles: death rates of children under 15: England and Wales.

Note that the graph from The Guardian starts almost at the very end of the above graph. It is debatable as to whether the vaccine had any effect on decreases in death rates, and obviously illogical in the extreme to assume that the declining trends occurring before vaccination would suddenly give way to an increase in levels if we stopped vaccinating; when asked to respond to this: **The Guardian declined to comment.**

4.1.1 Smallpox – eradication?

Turning to the story of smallpox vaccination, we see an almost blind faith and disregard of available evidence in the much-touted anecdote 'smallpox has been eradicated by vaccination'.

> ➤ In England free **smallpox vaccines were introduced in 1840** and made compulsory in 1853.
> ➤ Between 1857 and 1859 there were 14,244 deaths from smallpox. Between 1863 and 1865 after a population rise of 7%, the **death rate rose by 40.8%** to 20,059.
> ➤ In 1867 evaders of vaccination were prosecuted. Those left unvaccinated were very few. Between 1870 and 1872 after a population rise of 9%, the **death rate rose by 123%** to 44,840.
> ➤ Then we see the phenomena of reclassification, at the time all authorities agree that chickenpox is non-fatal. Yet in the 30 years up to 1934, 3,112 people are stated to have died of chickenpox and only 579 of smallpox in England and Wales.

Smallpox was the <u>first illness</u> to be targeted with a mass vaccination campaign in 1840, which in fact lead to a dramatic <u>increase in death rates</u> from smallpox when most other illnesses without vaccines were experiencing a steady decline.

(See the mortality rates of Scarlet fever, diphtheria, tuberculosis, whooping cough, tetanus and measles above).

When eventually mortality did decline, lagging behind all the other illnesses looked at, we are told that this was due to the highly successful smallpox vaccine; a conclusion that could only have been drawn by someone ignoring all the medical evidence to date.

Because levels of illness have been declining for many years prior to vaccination, evidently there are many factors responsible for this, other than the use of vaccines. So we are left with the issue of deciding what effect did vaccines have over and above what clearly would have happened anyway?

4.2 Reporting of illness

But even if levels of illness were consistent and unchanging prior to vaccines, we still have a potential problem with the accuracy of our figures. The problem that researchers face, (especially those studying the epidemiology of illnesses i.e. the incidence of illness in real populations), is the accuracy of the reporting. Are there factors that affect the actual reporting of disease?

Investigations do in fact confirm the phenomenon of under reporting illnesses in vaccinated individuals. Many cases of whooping cough which occur in vaccinated children would be subject to "re-diagnosis".

> *"Family doctors might tend to diagnose and notify whooping cough less often in immunized children than in un-immunized ones".*
>
> *Dr Norman Noah (BMJ 17/1/1976)*

> *"General Practitioners are much less likely to notify whooping cough in vaccinated children where the symptoms are typical. The figures may therefore underrate the incidence in vaccinated children".*
>
> *Professor Gordon Stewart (The Lancet 29/1/1977)*

> *Anthony Harnden in Oxford UK found that over a third of his study group of children presenting with a persistent cough had whooping cough, 85% had been fully immunised i.e. had all three booster shots of the whooping cough vaccine (therefore the 85% figure did not include those that had received one or two shots of whooping cough vaccine).*
>
> *Anthony Hamden et al, (BMJ 7/07/06)*

Doctors are therefore more likely to diagnose illnesses using a different name if a patient appears to be presenting symptoms of an illness that they have been vaccinated against. This is not a groundless cynicism but a real consequence of:

> ➢ The actual difficulty in deciding what illness somebody has, especially if it is mild and in the early stages.
> ➢ The difficulty in diagnosing illnesses that have become less common since the declines from the 1850's to the present day.
> ➢ The pressure to find appropriate treatment as quickly as possible and therefore the desire to eliminate unlikely diagnosis.
> ➢ The universal faith in vaccines and therefore the inherent bias that presents in diagnosing illness.

All of which creates a bias in favour of reporting a lower incidence of a particular illness after the introduction of its specific vaccine. Many people today have first hand experience of this phenomenon; for example when taking their children along to see their doctor with what they clearly see to be measles, they find their doctor unwilling to give a diagnosis as such because the child has previously been vaccinated against measles.

This documented and real bias in reporting does create a reduced incidence of illness after the introduction of a vaccine even if the actual incidence remains unchanged.

One interesting example of this can be illustrated by looking at an event that occurred in the USA. In 1982, a TV programme called "DPT - Vaccine Roulette" was screened highlighting the dangers of the Pertussin component of the DPT triple vaccine (the P part of DPT, the vaccination against whooping cough). Symptoms of neurological damage, including paralysis, epilepsy, brain damage and cot death were observed. As a result of this public viewing and increased public awareness of the possible dangers of the vaccine, the uptake of the vaccine fell and many more people chose not to vaccinate with DPT but with DT omitting the Pertussin component.

Consequently the incidence of whooping cough increased across America, but that is to say, the numbers of 'reported' cases were increasing. We were being told there were more cases of whooping cough, and epidemics were reported in at least two American States, Maryland and Wisconsin. This was of course blamed on the decline in whooping cough vaccine uptake. However Dr Anthony Morris an expert on bacterial and viral diseases and member of the FDA (the drugs licensing body in the USA) decided to investigate these cases of whooping cough through laboratory testing. In Maryland, 5 of the 41 cases were confirmed cases of whooping cough and in Wisconsin, 16 of the 43 cases were confirmed.

Dr Morris concluded that whooping cough cases were being <u>over reported</u> where <u>doctors expected</u> to see an increase in cases due to low vaccine uptake. Even more interesting was the finding that ALL confirmed cases of whooping cough occurred in individuals that <u>had been vaccinated.</u> Dr Morris further concluded that whooping cough cases were probably being under reported in vaccinated individuals, the diagnosis of whooping cough in these vaccinated cases would <u>not</u> have come to light in the absence of the whooping cough scare from the TV program and the subsequent investigation.

Here we have a documentary that was blamed for the reduced uptake of vaccines and consequently held responsible for the rise in whooping cough cases which was therefore used in subsequent media stories as the reason why we should vaccinate our children, when in fact the only children with whooping cough were those that were vaccinated.

The ineffectiveness of a vaccine was misrepresented by the media to actually promote the vaccine.

A similar story was perpetuated about a religious group in the Netherlands when an epidemic of polio was reported in 1992. The polio epidemic was blamed on the unvaccinated members of the religious group that do not believe in vaccinations. However the article in Morbidity Mortality and Weekly Report of the CDC 16/10/92 (41);775-778 showed that this epidemic consisted of only five people across the whole country in which none of the cases were epidemiologically linked and the two cases from the religious group that had supposedly started this epidemic had both been vaccinated with polio vaccine, one had been vaccinated just the day before.

> *News stories, albeit entertaining, do not provide a sound basis for anyone to make health choices.*

We also know there are other factors affecting the judgment of family doctors in the UK, since the 1990's these doctors have been given pay incentives to vaccinate a greater percentage of the population. In line with certain percentage vaccine uptake, the more they vaccinate the more money they earn, this has also met with publicly expressed criticism from doctors themselves and obviously puts pressure on them to promote vaccinations thereby overstating the benefits, understating and underreporting the problems.

The trust in such a system is further eroded when we are faced with an astonishing refusal to accept the basis of potential problems by government health advisors, ministers and policy makers. The following reply was sent to me personally in a letter from J. St.Juste of The Department of Health (4/02/92) in response to questions about the effects of pay incentives to doctors to vaccinate higher levels of the population:

> *"I should like to explain that doctors do not receive a higher income for carrying out childhood immunisation; they receive bonus payments on top of their pay for achieving high levels of immunisation."*

This double-speak and attempt at denial raises serious concerns as to the ability of the health department to openly inform the public of any problems that are associated with their health policies.

4.3 The classification of illness.

So far we have seen the dramatic effects of other health factors affecting the incidence of illness from the 1850's to 1950's and also how reporting bias can affect statistics; we shall now turn our attention to how illnesses are classified and the impact on disease numbers.

We have briefly discussed how infectious illnesses are classified, since the advent of germ theory the illness is labelled according to the microbe that is said to be responsible for the illness. If measles virus or the poliovirus is identified in an individual then the illness presenting will be classified accordingly, measles or polio. This may appear perfectly logical but as we shall see with regard to illnesses this does in fact add to our statistical conundrum.

The human body contains trillions of microbes that live normally within us, therefore the initial problem is to verify which microbe if any is the cause of the illness, finding illnesses **associated** with viruses, is not the same as determining that the virus was the cause. Then with the introduction of a medical procedure that appears to tackle a microbe, there is of course the danger that the susceptibility to the illness is not addressed and the initial microbe is simply replaced by another.

For example within the populations of viruses within the human body, the wild type polio viruses account for three of a family of 72 viruses, of which the remainder are not called polio viruses. In a person that develops paralysis, poliovirus may be found and we deem that to be the cause; developing a procedure that eradicates the poliovirus from others could equally leave them open to paralysis associated with other viruses, as is the case with paralysis associated with Echo or Coxsackie virus. It has also been reported (The Lancet, 1962:548-51) that diseases associated with these other viruses may be more severe than the illnesses associated with the poliovirus that they have replaced, and therefore, although the patient appears to have been prevented from contracting polio, they are now susceptible to more serious illnesses.

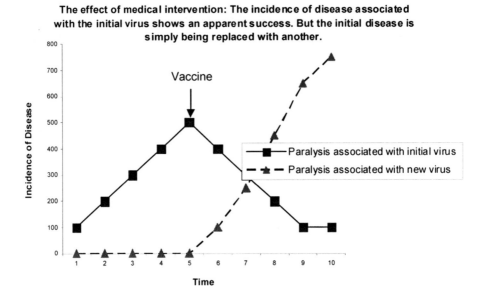

The effect of medical intervention: The incidence of disease associated with the initial virus shows an apparent success. But the initial disease is simply being replaced with another.

If we are to show the numbers of cases of paralytic disease associated with the initial virus on a graph, it will appear that the medical intervention has caused a reduced incidence of disease, but unless we see the incidence of all the associated illnesses we will not see the corresponding increase of the exact same illness associated with a slightly different form of the virus. The graph would appear to illustrate a successful medical intervention, but the actual disease susceptibility remains unaltered or possibly worsened, illness still persists in the population and as an individual you are no better off having paralysis associated with Echo virus than you are with polio virus.

One additional statistical manipulation that worked in favour of vaccine promoters was the re-classification of paralytic poliomyelitis. From 1955 in order to be suffering from paralytic poliomyelitis a patient had to exhibit symptoms of paralysis for 60 days. Prior to 1954 patients had to exhibit symptoms for only 24 hours, the polio vaccine was introduced in 1955, consequently **1000's of cases of polio were reduced to dozens** simply by changing the criteria of polio disease classification.

4.4 The classification of non-vaccinated

The failure of vaccines to protect or create a significant immune response according to the criteria of vaccine promoters has led to the need to revaccinate individuals, a phenomenon that doesn't exist with natural immunity. Once you contract measles naturally, for the vast majority, this would confer life-long immunity, however, many vaccines require additional 'boosters' and they are often spaced by a period of about a month or so and for some several years.

An individual is therefore <u>only fully vaccinated</u> after they have received <u>all boosters</u>. If three vaccines are required for a full course of treatment then after being vaccinated once or twice you are still classified as being 'not fully vaccinated'. However when comparing the incidence of disease in non-vaccinated and vaccinated, those that actually have been vaccinated but not 'fully vaccinated' can often be presented as non-vaccinated.

In a small percentage of the population, vaccines are known to cause the illness that you are being vaccinated against; this could be due to; a particularly problematic vaccine batch and/or an individual that is highly susceptible to the vaccine. If in a susceptible individual this does occur, then it is very likely to happen after just one vaccine. As a result of this, disease rates will actually appear to be higher in the so-called not fully vaccinated, even though it is actually being caused by the vaccine.

The incidence of illness in the not 'fully vaccinated' would actually be used as an argument by pro-vaccinators to justifying further use of the vaccine.

4.5 Shifting age groups

It is interesting to note that measles, mumps and rubella among vaccinated, and therefore supposedly immune, individuals continues to be reported. These diseases, which are essentially benign self-limiting diseases of childhood, are being diagnosed later in adolescents and adults, which are more severe, with complications that include liver abnormalities, pneumonia and arthritis.

If health authorities show a reduction in the numbers of cases of these illnesses in vaccinated children, (classically 0-15 years old), such studies would of course appear to show that the vaccine works in reducing the incidence of illness. However, if these vaccinated children go on to develop these illnesses later in adolescence and adulthood; we are of course not reducing illness just delaying them. Worse still these delayed illnesses may be more severe than if they had been contracted at a younger age, none of which would have been apparent if we confine our statistics to the 0-15 year olds.

4.6 Illness and whole people

We are all well aware of the fact that some illnesses are more serious than others; therefore with increased levels of health, within a given population, one would expect to see a decrease in numbers of individuals contracting illness as well as a decrease in severity of illnesses.

If on the other hand, after a given medical procedure, the incidence of a mild illness was to decrease, we could only be sure that this is a positive sign if it is not accompanied by an increase in more severe illnesses.

A graph showing the effects of thalidomide on nausea during pregnancy would show favourable results, a decrease in symptoms of nausea associated with use of the drug. However, as has been learnt to our cost in the 1960's and 1970's, the use of this drug was unfortunately accompanied by severe and irreversible abnormalities in the unborn child. Nevertheless according to the graphs, the drug was and is successful.

The introduction of Mumps vaccine could result in a lower incidence of mumps but the vaccine can also result in more serious problems such as mumps meningitis. If as a result of a vaccine children lose a susceptibility to one kind of mild illness but increase a susceptibility to a more severe illness, incidence graphs will still appear to show that the vaccine is successful.

These graphs do not illustrate what happens to real people in real situations, in order to make an assessment of the best way forward regarding any therapeutic intervention we need to know what happens as a result of that treatment to the whole person over an extended period of time. Amputations below the knee will reduce the number of ankle injuries among children, but at what cost? In our assessment of treatment, it is not acceptable to ignore this question and it is no more complicated than that.

4.7 The numbers

The problems highlighted above increase in significance when we start to appreciate the low percentages involved regarding the incidence of infectious illnesses within any given population. For example, a polio epidemic is of the order of 35 per 100,000 and before 1955 was 20 per 100,000. Small reporting and statistical errors can have huge implications.

Note in the MMR vaccine example already mentioned, mumps meningitis a known side effect of the vaccine, was thought to be occurring at acceptably low levels (1 in 143,000). However, after years of MMR use and only after reported problems in Canada did the UK health authorities carry out more detailed studies. It was then found that the MMR vaccine was causing mumps meningitis in as much as1 in 4,000 patients. Therefore it was possible to create more problems than were being solved, causing almost epidemic proportions of mumps meningitis, equating to 25 in 100,000, without the medical profession even noticing.

Members of the general public are often surprised at the small percentages involved in so-called epidemics, it is therefore more difficult than people realise to get a true picture of illnesses within the population and it is something that remains outside of the experience of most of us, including family doctors. With a maximum patient list of between 2 to 3,000, within a local area most doctors would be likely to see between 1 to 2 patients with the epidemic illness, assuming that everyone with the illness has been to see their doctor. We simply do not have sufficient overview, and consequently we are vulnerable to being sold anything as the 'truth'. The epidemic figures of the 1850's do not apply to the era of our vaccines apart from the smallpox vaccine.

We are in the midst of an epidemic of acquired immune deficiency disease, autoimmune disease, allergies and autism, all of which continue to rise, are we aware of this scenario? In order to find answers to the question of safety and effectiveness of any medical intervention, especially that of vaccines, where we cannot immediately see their effects, we have to delve a little below the surface. It is not enough to rely on graphs showing disease notifications and certainly misleading to rely on the reports of the media.

Epidemics and the dangers of disease may sound frightening, and vaccines eradicating illness may appear significant, until we see how low these figures are and realise that our knowledge actually comes from statistical analysis. Statistical analysis based on reports that are fraught with inaccuracies, analysed by personnel with inherent bias and uncertainty, because, at best, the impact of vaccines has been minimal, the dangers underestimated and therefore it is actually impossible to see from an individual's experience whether vaccines are of benefit or detriment.

We are given the impression that 1000's of people died of illnesses in epidemics across the globe, until vaccines came along to save us all, vaccines that we are told were responsible for dramatic reductions in disease. This has actually <u>never</u> been the case; the vast majority of the reductions in disease came well BEFORE the introduction of vaccines and these age-old vaccines have a reputation that may be entirely due to improvements in living conditions.

4.8 Comparison of vaccinated and non-vaccinated

> *"If your experiment needs statistics, you ought to have done a better experiment."*

Ernest Rutherford
The father of Nuclear Physics, Nobel Prize for Chemistry 1908

It is common in research that promotes vaccines, to quote death rates and disease statistics in individuals that are at the lower end of the social scale and compare with vaccinated individuals at the higher end.

This will obviously create an overestimate of the benefit of vaccines because the vaccinated group is naturally healthier regardless of their vaccination. This research bias has been known throughout the ages but is still a common feature in vaccine statistics.

George Bernard Shaw's extracts from the preface to his play entitled
'The Doctor's Dilemmas'

Public ignorance of the laws of evidence and of statistics can hardly be exaggerated. ... apparently overwhelming statistical evidence in favour of any preventative can be produced by persuading the public that everybody caught the disease formerly.

Thus if a disease is one which normally attacks fifteen per cent of the population, and if the effect of a preventative is actually to increase the proportion to twenty percent, the publication of this figure of twenty per cent will convince the public that the preventative has reduced the percentage by eighty per cent instead of increasing it by five, because the public, left to itself and to the old gentlemen who are always ready to remember, on every possible subject, that things used to be much worse than they are now, will assume that the former was about 100 percent.

The vogue of the Pasteur treatment of hydrophobia (rabies), for instance, was due to the assumption by the public that every person bitten by a rabid dog necessarily got rabies. I myself heard rabies discussed in my youth by doctors in Dublin before a Pasteur Institute existed, the subject having been brought forward there by the scepticism of an eminent surgeon as to whether rabies is really a specific disease or only ordinary tetanus induced (as Tetanus was then supposed to be induced) by a lacerated wound. There were no statistics available as to the proportion of dog bites that ended in rabies; but nobody ever guessed that the cases could be more than two or three per cent of the bites.

... It seemed to me that the proportion of deaths among the cases treated at the (Pasteur) Institute was rather higher, if anything, than might have been expected had there been no Institute in existence. But to the public every Pasteur patient who did not die was miraculously saved from an agonising death by the beneficent white magic of that most trusty of all wizards, the man of science...

...In the case of a preventative enforced by law, this illusion is intensified grotesquely, because only vagrants can evade it. Now vagrants have little power of resisting any disease: their death rate and their case-mortality rate are always high relative to that of respectable folk. Nothing is easier, therefore, than to prove that compliance with any public regulation produces the most gratifying results. It would be equally easy even if the regulation actually raised the death-rate, provided it did not raise it sufficiently to make the average householder, who cannot evade regulations, die as early as the average vagrant who can.

For example in 'The Journal of Infectious Disease' (01/02/00 Vol.181, B.I.Niyazmatov et al) comparisons are made between vaccinated and non-vaccinated at the time of the Soviet Union collapse in 1990 when facilities went into decline and certain families could not gain access to vaccines, therefore this became one of the very rare opportunities to compare vaccinated and non-vaccinated. However the main reason for the emergence of a non-vaccinated group of individuals was their lack of finances, isolation and inability to access health facilities i.e. those people at the very lowest end of the economic ladder. This non-vaccinated group cannot be compared to vaccinated individuals at the higher socio-economic end, the obvious bias in analysis when comparing these two groups is completely omitted in the paper's discussion and so we see that poor evidence showing apparent effectiveness of vaccines is wholeheartedly embraced in spite of such glaring inaccuracies.

However evidence showing vaccines in a less favourable light is treated somewhat differently. For example Ines Kristensen, Peter Aaby, and Henrik Jensen, published research in BMJ 9/12/00, (321:1435) showing that DPT and polio vaccines were associated with increased death rates in children.

> "… recipients of one dose of diphtheria, tetanus, and pertussis or polio vaccines had **higher mortality** (death rate) than children who had received none of these vaccines"

This research was of course very important in looking at the wider effects of vaccines other than their ability to produce antibodies or their impact on only one specific disease, <u>surprisingly this kind of research is very rarely carried out</u>. The following comments were written by Professor Kim Mulholland and Professor Mauricio L Barreto, who were requested by the WHO, to visit Guinea-Bissau during 8-15 October 2000 to review this study.

> *"Regardless of the outcome of the ongoing investigations, the work in Guinea-Bissau highlights the importance of considering the overall impact of vaccines on children's health...*
>
> *Broader lessons can be learnt from this study. Public health research to support public health interventions is not a luxury but a necessity. Up till now, the overall impact of routine childhood vaccines on survival in places with high mortality has __not__ yet been evaluated systematically. We should learn from this omission and ensure that all public health interventions are underpinned by the appropriate public health research, both experimental and observational, to ensure that they are both safe and efficacious."*
>
> BMJ 10/02/2001;322:360

The results caused a certain alarm with the WHO and other vaccine promoters. However, the same study showed that BCG and measles vaccine groups appeared to survive longer than unvaccinated groups and therefore the WHO and others were happy to proclaim that these vaccines promote longevity even though this was not due to preventing measles or TB deaths, i.e. in ways that are not explained by the vaccine.

In response to the negative finding on DPT the WHO commissioned further investigations but was of course happy with the BCG and measles vaccine conclusion even though these results were not in keeping with the effects of the vaccines and were of course subject to potential bias as the original research states:

> *"Vaccinated children had more contact with the health system, their mothers being more likely to have received tetanus vaccination during pregnancy and to have given birth outside the home. Vaccinated children had larger arm circumference and their mothers tended to be younger and have fewer children, to have a latrine in their compound,*

> *Since children weighing less than 2500 g are not supposed to receive BCG, unvaccinated children could represent a negatively selected group"*

Aaby & Jensen BMJ 9/12/00 (321:1435)

These factors should of course lead one to view the results with some skepticism, in fact given the likelihood of a selection bias towards a better health group in those vaccinated (greater access to health care, toilets, higher birth weight etc) the results may have reduced the apparent benefit of BCG and increased the number of deaths in the DPT group.

> *If one believes that mothers complying with the vaccination programme have children with lower mortality, the beneficial effect of BCG and measles may have been overestimated whereas the harmful effect of diphtheria, tetanus, pertussis and polio vaccines would have been underestimated.*

Aaby & Jensen BMJ response 10/01/01

However, it was of course the DPT results that were most alarming because these were undermining the value of the vaccine policy of the WHO and in fact most of the vaccine policies around the world. In response, the WHO commissioned several follow-up studies and found that this negative DPT effect could only be found in this study in Guinea-Bissau. However using the analysis of these new WHO studies Aaby and Jensen found that their own results would also appear to show NO negative effect of the DPT and polio vaccines, could there be something wrong with the analysis?

There were of course problems with these follow-up studies, as Aaby and Jensen of the original study describe in the BMJ response entitled ***"DTP in low income countries: improved child survival or survival bias?"*** 9/04/05 (330:845-846). The WHO commissioned studies had one glaringly obvious methodological error:

"When a child dies, the vaccination card is usually thrown away; and information on vaccination is therefore collected conditionally on survival to the subsequent visit. **If an unvaccinated child was vaccinated and died before the next visit the death would be classified as unvaccinated...** *Such survival bias may turn a negative estimate into a positive one: our original 84% increase in mortality for one dose of DTP became a 32% reduction"*

The WHO however accepted the results of these trials even though a huge inaccuracy existed and as typified by vaccine promoters are generally happy to accept sloppy methodology in the promotion of vaccines but criticise more rigorous studies if they illustrate the harmful effects of vaccines. Of course what is needed are <u>properly</u> controlled trials, trials that the vaccine community say we have, however Paul E M Fine, (Professor of communicable disease epidemiology London School of Hygiene and Tropical Medicine) obviously thinks otherwise in commenting on the above studies:

"These studies faced very difficult methodological challenges and have been unable convincingly to get round the obvious huge confounding associated with the selective distribution of vaccines. Given that confounding, the only way rigorously to study such outcomes is by **trials.**"

Yet from the studies available, the WHO feel confident in promoting vaccines and their ability to reduce death rates, even though this is not supported by the available data:

"In modelling exercises, vaccination against diphtheria, pertussis, tetanus, and polio has been **assumed to save 1.5-2.0% of the children** *in areas with high infant mortality. However,* **these assumptions are not supported by data,** *and few studies of the effect of routine vaccinations other than*

measles on mortality have been carried out in developing countries".

Aaby and Jensen – BMJ 9/12/00

With all of these factors taken into account; declines in incidence of illness due to factors other than vaccination, reporting bias, classification changes of disease, inappropriate comparisons of vaccinated and non-vaccinated, focus on antibody production and not the actual incidence of illness and death, and we then add this to the facts outlined by Antonio Coutinho, Director of Immunology Research at institutes in France and Portugal, where he states that:

"...Centuries after Jenner's 'vaccination' and more than 100 years after Louis Pasteur's principle of 'attenuated' vaccines, we are still totally devoid of vaccines against chronic infections and against a large number of acute infections. Several decades of 'DNA technology' and 'biotechnology' have failed to produce all the new effective, 'no-risk' vaccines we expected. Most vaccines used today are of the 'conventional' type, many of which were discovered when we had little knowledge of immunology, and absolutely no information on the cells and molecules of the immune system. Obviously, the lack of clinical success means that our understanding of the immune system, despite decades of intense research, still remains elusive..."

European Molecular Biology Organisation (EMBO) Reports (2003)

We see that very few new vaccines have since been produced, and given the massive reductions in disease that had happened before vaccines were introduced the effects of the old vaccines are at best minimal. It is in this light we begin to see that the role of vaccines in disease prevention is in fact highly questionable and in desperate need of rigorous trials.

4.9 To summarise

Given the above confounding factors, it would appear to be very difficult to assess the effects of vaccines simply by looking at the incidence of reported illnesses in the population and charting those in the form of a graph; such information leaves many more questions unanswered.

> ➢ We know that factors other than vaccination have had the greater influence on health and illness over the last century and therefore we need to separate those effects from that of vaccines. It is possible that vaccines have had little or no effect at all but may appear to improve health and reduce disease due to the backdrop of decline that occurs as a result of improvements in standards of living.
> ➢ Classification of illness and consequently reporting before and after vaccinations are not consistent, this needs to be standardised before and after the introduction of a vaccine in order to make worthwhile comparisons.
> ➢ We need to take into account the effects of the vaccine on the whole person and observe what other systems in the body are being affected before we can even say that a reduction in incidence of one illness is necessarily a good thing.
> ➢ It is vital to systematically screen for symptoms before and after vaccines rather than wait for members of the public to report symptoms to their doctors, who then have to decide whether or not to report the incident to the health authority as vaccine related. We therefore need to make observations over months and years, after a vaccine is introduced rather than being influenced by the legal time restrictions of 72 hours or 14 days, when deciding how safe and effective a vaccine is.
> ➢ In developing countries the unvaccinated are people with less access to health services generally and with low standards of living so cannot be compared to vaccinated individuals that are healthier due to other factors.
> ➢ Vaccine trials are conducted on healthy people; adverse effects to illnesses tend to happen in those that are already very sick,

comparing risk of vaccine to risk of illness in this manner is therefore unscientific and substantially biased.

These are fundamental medical principles and the fact that they have not been addressed positions the evidence of pro-vaccinators in a very poor and unscientific light. It appears to place the burden of proof on to the general public, so that members of the lay community have been left to research and decide whether vaccines are safer and more effective than natural immunity.

We have looked at the historical anecdotes of those in favour of vaccination, the arguments based on antibody levels, the incidence and death rates of disease in the population over time, plus comparisons of vaccinated individuals in developing countries with those that were not vaccinated. All of these studies were however lacking in credibility and in fact seemed to suggest that there were more important factors other than vaccination responsible for declines in disease rates and that the actual dangers of vaccines are being systematically overlooked; is it possible to design trials that could overcome these limitations?

4.10 Vaccine trials.

It is relatively easy to design trials that would establish much more accurately than the graphs presented by the UK Health Authorities whether in fact vaccines work and at what price to our health.

In principle how could we test a vaccine? Very simply, we would have to vaccinate a group of people and compare them to a non-vaccinated group. In designing such a trial we would also need to take into account the effect of telling volunteers of the trial whether or not they were to be vaccinated.

In one particular documented example in a military hospital during World War II, as would often happen during times of heavy casualties, the American anaesthetist Henry Beecher ran out of morphine and was in a dilemma as to whether to carry out the operation, even if potentially successful the procedure could send the patient into fatal shock. This was the only painkilling drug available to anaesthetise soldiers with severe injuries and for use during emergency surgical operations; however the physician noticed something incredible, a nurse injected his patient with saline solution (salt solution) instead. Amazingly the saline solution worked, it was producing remarkable pain-killing effects, even though the chemical properties of saline do not act as a painkiller.

Believing they were being injected with a powerful painkiller, patients allowed their own healing process to take effect; this is known as the 'placebo' effect. Here the healing effect is not due to the chemical action of the drug but the healing ability of the patient that has been stimulated by the thought of taking what they believe to be a powerful and healing drug.

This is in fact quite conceivable in normal medical terms, given that the body's own natural painkillers are actually more powerful than morphine. However in a trauma situation most individuals would react with fear and panic, which seriously impairs their own healing process, making it necessary to intervene with powerful medication.

If vaccines were considered to be beneficial, members of the vaccinated group would consider themselves fortunate and this could have a positive effect on their health, the 'placebo' effect, this positive effect due to the belief of the patient in the treatment would occur whether in fact the vaccine works or not. This placebo effect is actually very powerful, just as the negative effect on patients receiving no vaccine, if of course they believed the vaccine to be beneficial.

Therefore in order to distinguish the effect of the vaccine from that of placebo, a trial would have to be a 'blind' placebo controlled trial. All participants of the trial would be subjected to a similar procedure, some would be administered the real vaccine and others a placebo, (placebo containing no active vaccine) and none of them would be told whether or not they are receiving the real vaccine or the placebo.

Interestingly in the example above, the first signs of the salt solution failure, (placebo failure), occurred when the staff administering the injections realised they were giving salt solution instead of morphine. As a result it has become a well-known medical phenomenon that the thoughts and beliefs of the practitioner administering the placebo can have a considerable impact on the effect of the placebo response. Consequently trials are designed whereby the personnel administering the procedure as well as the patients are unaware of whether they are using placebo or real drug. Therefore such trials are called 'double-blind' placebo-controlled trials.

One more factor that needs to be taken into account is the method by which the two groups are chosen. The placebo group and the vaccinated group have to be sufficiently large enough to be statistically significant and they need to be similar. It would be no good comparing a group of people in one town of one country to a group in a different town of another country, each having different geographical, economic and social conditions. One way to ensure similarity and no prejudice in sampling would be to have a 'random' choice of placebo and vaccinated from the <u>same</u> population in a given geographical area.

We would now have our 'randomised double-blind placebo-controlled trial'. This is in fact a very common method of assessing the effectiveness of almost <u>all</u> pharmaceutical drugs, it is not always suitable for all medical procedures, those involving; surgery, counseling, bodywork and any procedure with high patient therapist interaction, and highly individualised treatment. Such procedures can be tested, but the trials have to be suitably designed.

Vaccines are the same for all recipients they are not individualised according to the patient, they are used as preventatives (prophylaxis), they are not used to treat something that already exists in a patient and therefore the patient cannot readily see if the vaccine works. Even without vaccinations the numbers of people that will contract many of these diseases are very low compared to those that will never contract the illness.

Vaccines are also given because they are said to reduce the severity of an illness. Even if you were to contract the Illness that you have been vaccinated against, vaccine promoters say that the illness will be less severe than if you had not been vaccinated. Thereby vaccines are said to reduce the incidence and severity of illness. For the most part we are therefore comparing the severity of an illness in vaccinated to the severity of illness in non-vaccinated. Remembering that at any one time, even during an epidemic, there are as little as 35 people in 100,000 with the illness. Severity is often measured in death rates; vaccines are often promoted on the basis of reducing death rates and deaths would therefore be much less frequent than the incidence of 35 in 100,000.

Deaths from measles had reduced from 1200 per million in the 1850's to about 6 in the 1950's before the vaccine was even introduced and showed every sign of reducing further still, as did deaths from scarlet fever without the use of a vaccine. Deaths due to scarlet fever dropped from 2,250 per million in the 1850s to zero in the 1950's and has remained so even though there has never been a vaccine for scarlet fever.

Consequently there are many difficulties to overcome when assessing the effectiveness and safety of vaccines; this cannot be accurately evaluated by simply adding up numbers of cases reported by doctors to the various health authorities and then plotting this on a graph. It is essential that large-scale placebo-controlled trials of vaccines be carried out, as is the case with almost all other pharmaceutical drugs.

In fact many people even within the medical profession think that these trials are carried out, Andrew Blann, a virologist, found the criticisms of vaccination in my previous book hard to accept. He stated that the medical community knows that the benefits of vaccines outweigh the disadvantages because …"If you take 2000 people in danger of infection, and vaccinate half, there will be fewer infections in those immunized". Effectively he was stating, in a confident, 'matter of fact' manner that the placebo-control trials that we carry out for vaccines show that they are safe and effective.

However, probably to his surprise and on further questioning, he failed to produce details of a single trial that had been carried out in that most basic manner, simply comparing half of the members of a group that had been vaccinated with another half that had not.

The question of placebo-controlled trials in their most basic form has been presented to vaccine producers in the UK. They say unfortunately that they have none. In fact vaccine producers are not required to produce a single placebo controlled trial in order to introduce a vaccine into the population, a vaccine that would be subsequently injected into a small child or adult.

In questioning why, it is often stated that such trials would be unethical. Which is an interesting stance considering that almost all other pharmaceutical drugs have to be tested in this way.

4.10.1 Why are 'placebo controlled trials' considered unethical?

The current medical establishment have very little to offer in the way of treatment for most infectious diseases, they say the best way to deal with them is by preventing them from occurring in the first place through the use of vaccines. Therefore withholding vaccines from half of your test group, to create a placebo group, would be denying them medical care, even though the vaccine may not be 100% safe or effective, consequently any such trial would be deemed unethical. The implication therefore is that vaccines are more effective and are safer than natural immunity and that they don't need such rigorous testing.

This is of course a way of denying that any problems exist with vaccines that could in fact outweigh any benefit, therefore any possible benefit from vaccines is bound to be better than nothing. The benefit of vaccinating an individual is often compared in principle to an unprotected individual, which somehow assumes that without vaccines we have no immunity, which is of course medical nonsense. Vaccine trials are only unethical if we <u>know</u> that any benefit over and above our natural immunity <u>outweighs</u> any adverse effect and how do we know that unless we conduct proper trials? It is of course a convenient circular reasoning, that is however, not shared by all within the medical profession. The Cochrane Collaboration was set up in 1992 by the UK National Health Service Research and Development Program to assess trials published in peer reviewed scientific journals, the head of the Vaccines Division is Tom Jefferson, writing in the British Medical Journal he states:

> "The inception of a vaccination campaign seems to preclude the assessment of a vaccine through placebo controlled randomised trials on ethical grounds. Far from being unethical, however, such trials are desperately needed and we should invest in them without delay. A further consequence is reliance on non-randomised studies once the campaign is under way. It is debatable whether these can contribute to our understanding of the effectiveness of vaccines."
>
> BMJ (28/10/06; 333: 912-915)

4.10.2 The Placebo Injustice

Interestingly, if after conducting a placebo controlled trial it transpires that the placebo is better than the vaccine, we would then be obliged to carry out a trial to compare placebo against doing nothing. Remember placebo is giving somebody a dummy pill that they think is effective against a condition, this may or may not be better than doing nothing at all. If there is no difference between giving placebo and doing nothing, we can assume the placebo fared better in the vaccine trial due to the side-effects and therefore the downside of the vaccine, consequently we are better off not using that particular vaccine.

If however we find that the placebo is better than doing nothing, which is possible given the nature of placebo and the power of mind in disease, we may consider that we would be duty bound to give placebo to our patients, it would in fact be unethical not to carry out a mass immunisation campaign using placebo, given that it is the best intervention that we have and actually better than doing nothing. Of course we rarely do trial the placebo in such a way, possibly so that we can avoid such moral and commercial dilemmas, nevertheless the issue of ethics does weigh heavily in favour of conducting placebo controlled trials rather than not.

A search through vaccine literature will reveal references to many placebo controlled trials, so what exactly are we saying here? These trials are either placebo controlled trials to assess immunogenicity, that is, tests to find out if the vaccines work in producing antibodies, which isn't a trial to assess how the vaccine does in reducing severity or incidence of disease or they are trials comparing people vaccinated with various components of vaccines to other people vaccinated with other components of the vaccine. There are very few real placebo controlled trials, that is, unvaccinated without <u>any</u> of the harmful components of the vaccine therefore using some inert solution compared to vaccinated, because that is believed to be unethical.

4.10.3 Results of a placebo controlled vaccine trial

In spite of the reluctance to conduct placebo control trials, the results of one such trial were reported in the Lancet Jan 12 1980. The vaccine reviewed was the BCG vaccine, the vaccination against tuberculosis. It reported that although the protective efficacy of BCG was not rigorously assessed, the vaccine was increasingly used in Europe in the 1920's.

However, between 10/12/29 and 30/4/30, 251 of 412 infants born in Lübeck, Germany, received three doses of BCG vaccine during the first ten days of life. Of these 251, 72 died of tuberculosis within a few months of vaccination as a result of which the first well controlled trials of BCG were organized. There were 20 years of trials that followed, from 1935 to 1955, unfortunately the results of these trials were far from consistent, in fact The Lancet report states that, "their results varied strikingly and mysteriously", from 0% to 80%. Some trials concluded that the vaccine had no effect on the incidence of tuberculosis at all, with other trials showing a range of effectiveness from little more than 0% to as much as 80%.

Consequently in the 1970's the **largest placebo controlled field trial** ever carried out on the BCG vaccine was organised, with 260,000 participants, comparing equal sized vaccine and placebo control (non-vaccinated) groups. Not only did the results show **no evidence of a protective effect**, but slightly **more tuberculosis cases appeared in vaccinated** than in the equal sized placebo control group.

Therefore the most significant placebo controlled trial actually shows that individuals are more likely to get the illness if they were vaccinated. Of course something of a surprise, however what is even more damning was the lack of follow-up trials that should have followed swiftly after, trying to ascertain whether this was a problem of the trial or news of a vaccine that does not work. Although vaccine producers say they always try to improve on vaccines, the undeniable fact was that the most significant tuberculosis vaccine trial actually demonstrated that you were more likely to contract tuberculosis once you had been vaccinated, yet the vaccination continued in spite of this.

In a filmed debate in the Southampton UK 1995, the Head of the Pasteur Institute stated, in response to these criticisms: "Vaccines are not perfect but are better than nothing!" I was also a panel member at this debate and reminded him, that with regard to BCG, as determined by their own trials this was demonstrably NOT better than nothing, whereupon he eventually conceded that there were problems that were not addressed.

There appears to be a deep-seated conviction in the virtue of vaccines that dramatically affects the ability of researchers to assess the evidence rationally. This can be further illustrated by looking at the report published in 1993 by the US National Academy of sciences in which the American Academy of Paediatrics reaffirmed "Its long standing belief that the benefits of vaccines far outweigh the risks."

However, Russell Alexander a panel member and professor of epidemiology at the University of Washington, says he is disappointed that the panel did not compare the risk of vaccination with the risk of going unvaccinated. How was it therefore possible to come to the conclusion that "…the benefits of vaccines far outweigh the risks"? The benefit of a procedure is a statement of advantage over another procedure, or the advantage over not carrying out the procedure at all. Since there was no comparison of immunisation with another procedure, or with being unimmunised, the conclusions of the American Academy of Paediatrics are not based on scientific reasoning and are in fact meaningless.

Therefore the question of ethics and placebo-controlled trials seems to be turning on its head.

> There is evidence of the considerable effect of natural immunity: Over 95% reductions in mortality from measles, diphtheria, whooping cough, tuberculosis and tetanus before vaccines introduced. Scarlet fever the infectious illness causing the largest number of childhood deaths in 19th century UK diminished to zero before a vaccine was ever created. Therefore the ethical question remains do vaccines work over and above the effects of natural immunity; it is not a question of comparing vaccinated with unprotected, because natural immunity is a biological phenomenon that exists.

> Vaccines have also been produced that have later been found to be ineffective and consequently withdrawn. After many years of use, the cholera vaccine was withdrawn, with a statement from the World Health Organisation (WHO) recognising the need for safe clean water and proper waste disposal in preventing cholera epidemics, not the use of cholera vaccine.

> Vaccines have been produced that were later found to be causing more problems than they were solving. The mumps

component of the MMR vaccine (previously mentioned) was eventually found to be causing mumps encephalitis and was eventually withdrawn.

➢ Finally, the largest placebo-control trial on BCG vaccine against tuberculosis proved that you were more likely to get tuberculosis if you had been vaccinated.

➢ The harmful effects of vaccines are real, underestimated and very difficult to assess if we are vaccinating virtually everybody. This is why it takes so much work and concerted effort to assess the true effects of vaccines once they have become public health policy.

Therefore the current position of conducting no placebo control trials because it is unethical... is in itself unethical.

A placebo-controlled trial would be testing natural immunity against that of vaccinated individuals, to question the ethics involved in testing a vaccine against an 'unprotected person' presupposes that the vaccine protects, it also presupposes that without a vaccine one is unprotected, the conclusion is already in the question, a very confused way of avoiding the real question. Any individual alive and breathing has natural immunity, it is this you would be testing the vaccine against and it is this that vaccine promoters are reluctant to do.

CHAPTER FIVE

5 Is the Herd Immunity argument simply an emotional weapon to manipulate questioning parents?

Not content to give up responsibility for their health, people now wanted to blame others for their disease.

Those choosing not to vaccinate have often been accused of putting other people at risk of disease, by reducing 'herd immunity' and thus allowing the illness to propagate in the community. The unvaccinated would in theory jeopardise the health of those that were too ill to be vaccinated, by increasing the risk of passing the illness on to them. This does of course hinge on the assumption that vaccines work, and that vaccines do not in fact <u>increase illness</u> in the population.

It is of course an emotional and guilt laden attack on those choosing to address health issues other than by means of vaccination. But is a completely self-contained circular argument that negates to acknowledge that those choosing not to vaccinate do so from the conclusion that there are more effective ways of reducing disease in individuals and ultimately in the whole population, other than vaccination.

Because likewise if vaccines do not work then it is the vaccinated that are increasing illness in the population and it is the unvaccinated through obtaining long-lasting natural immunity that are reducing illness, protecting the health of themselves and ultimately the whole population. But let us indulge in the theory for a moment and ask what exactly, is 'herd immunity'?

5.1 Herd Immunity – The theory

Vaccine promoters and conventional medics from the perspective of germ theory and their newly acquired vaccines had a basis for developing further theories of epidemiology, and duly created models that they hoped could predict the incidence and severity of disease in vaccinated and unvaccinated populations. From an orthodox perspective the 'disease' was now a manifest externalised entity, pathogens exist and multiply within the patient and can be passed on to other susceptible individuals thereby spreading disease from person to person.

It had been observed that if the incidence of a disease naturally falls below a certain threshold it continued to decline making subsequent epidemics less likely. Declines in incidence were thought to be as a result of the increase in natural immunity through the process of having the illness, it was therefore postulated that the illness could further decline and indeed could be completely eradicated if the percentage of those immune reached above a certain threshold. The remaining susceptible individuals would not contract the disease because there were insufficient people to transmit the disease agent to them. According to this theory, sufficient numbers of immune individuals could result in the elimination of the disease for ever and this phasing out of the disease could actually occur before all people had the illness and therefore before all were immune. The immunity of the majority group, the 'herd immunity', would protect the others as a result of what became known as the 'herd effect'.

> *"Survival of the (disease) agent is crucial—if it cannot survive, it cannot invade and infect new hosts, and the epidemic ends."*

Epidemic theory –'The Encyclopaedia of public Health'

Assuming that vaccines can do the job of natural immunity, researchers in the nineteenth and twentieth century, William Farr, William Hamer, Ronald Ross, A. Hedrich, Fox, and others, superimposed mathematical formulae onto vaccine uptake figures to estimate what percentage of vaccine coverage in a given population would be necessary to create sufficient 'herd immunity' and thereby eliminate a disease, consequently protecting those not immune by this 'herd effect'.

5.2 Controversy

The concept is however controversial even within vaccine proponents of the scientific community, and yet many vaccine supporters speak of the 'herd effect' as though it was an absolute fact.

> "Several authors have written of data on measles which "challenge" the principle of herd immunity and others cite widely divergent estimates (from 70 to 95 percent) of the magnitude of the herd immunity threshold required for measles eradication. Still other authors have commented on the failure or "absence" of herd immunity against rubella and diphtheria. Authorities continue to argue over the extent to which different types of polio vaccine can, let alone do, induce herd immunity."

> Paul E.M. Fine Epidemiologic Reviews 1993
> The Johns Hopkins University, Vol. 15, No. 2

The mathematical models designed to predict the threshold of herd immunity to give a herd effect and thus eradicate an illness are however based on many oversimplifications: Firstly the numbers of susceptible individuals are taken to be everyone in the population that is either not vaccinated or not had the illness. There is the underlying assumption that _if_ one has not been vaccinated or had not naturally contracted the illness, then you were necessarily susceptible and therefore it was a matter of time before you would contract the disease given sufficient exposure to someone with the disease.

The rate of transmission although different for different illnesses was a fixed property that did not change over time, catching an illness was no more complicated than catching a ball and you would get no better at catching it over time or no worse, the probability of catching an illness was simply a property of the amount of people around you with sufficient balls for you to be able to catch one.

In addition, some estimates assumed that people intermingled completely randomly and that illness was not influenced by age, sex, socio-economic group, or season. Other models do make allowances for these factors but were modelled on closed systems with nobody coming into or out of the community, dying or being born. However when models started to approximate to real life scenarios things became rather more complicated.

More fundamentally the models do not take into account other known factors of disease:

> Clearly not everyone is susceptible to contracting a particular disease and may never be susceptible for the duration of their entire life; they will be neither vaccinated nor will they have contracted the illness naturally. For example, most people are exposed to, and naturally harbour, meningococcal bacteria and because a vaccine has only recently been introduced, most people alive today have never been vaccinated, yet most will never contract meningococcal meningitis, plainly we are not all susceptible. Therefore there is no uniformity of susceptibility as assumed by these models, the vast majority of people are not susceptible to these illnesses and only a fraction of a percentage are, and they are susceptible for very specific reasons.

> The mathematical models suggest a requirement to revaccinate populations because of the increase in numbers of susceptible individuals that are newly born, however these are the only sub-group of people classified as 'newly susceptible', omitting the complication of travellers in and out of communities. But additionally it implies that susceptibility to a disease cannot be newly acquired for other reasons. For

example individuals may become more susceptible over time due to other illnesses, or as a result of changes in lifestyle, trauma, medication, etc, similarly individuals may become less susceptible because of other improved health factors, these changes in susceptibility are not factored in to these mathematical equations.

The basic premise of herd immunity and therefore the consequent 'herd effect' also relies on the following assumptions:

➢ That any disease is primarily caused by only <u>one</u> specific microbe and that an effective vaccine against that microbe can in principle eliminate the 'disease'. However illnesses are in fact associated with any number of possible microbes and therefore a patient's disease is the result of the patient's specific susceptibility:

> *In many instances of illnesses that are clinically indistinguishable from paralytic poliomyelitis, polioviruses are not present. We therefore have acute paralytic diseases that have been renamed according to the presence of these other viruses, e.g. coxsackie viral paralysis, and echo viral paralysis.*
>
> The Lancet, 1962:548-51

➢ These mathematical models also assume that disease declines primarily as a result of immunity in the patient from either contracting the illness or being vaccinated, however vaccine promoters know that other changes in environmental conditions are also responsible for changes in incidence of disease, therefore disease can decrease for reasons other than herd immunity and herd effect.

> *The cholera vaccine was one of the first vaccines acknowledged to not impact on disease rates if the conditions of sanitation and clean drinking water were*

> *not addressed, consequently the vaccine was*
> *withdrawn.*

This is further demonstrated by the fact that as the disease conditions return the illnesses return, even in the vaccinated.

> *"… Russia made massive strides in arresting the spread of*
> *infectious diseases from 1970's to 1990. But the health status*
> *of the Russian population declined precipitously following the*
> *collapse of the Soviet Union in late 1991 with the concomitant*
> *decline in basic living conditions. Epidemics in the early 1990s*
> *caused diphtheria to increase 54-fold and the mortality rate to*
> *increase 35-fold. Further, there has been increased incidence*
> *of numerous other diseases that were earlier under control,*
> *including cholera, typhus, typhoid, whooping cough, measles,*
> *and hepatitis."*

> 'Health care systems in transition' Tragakes & Lessof
> Pub. The European Observatory on Health Systems & Policies

Many blame the epidemics on the fall in vaccine uptake rates evident with diphtheria for example since 1993, but much of the disease cases were between 1990 and 1996 and therefore only those under two or three years old would have been affected by the low vaccine rates since 1993. Most people born before 1990 would have been vaccinated, yet as illustrated in 'The Journal of Infectious Disease' (01/02/00 Vol.181, B.I.Niyazmatov et al) the epidemics affected mainly older people with the 0-2 year olds accounting for only 3.3% of the 1,227 cases.

Clearly given that vaccine status was a relatively constant feature for 20 years prior to the 1990 social collapse, it was in fact the dramatic declines in standards of living that were the major impetus to the resurgence of disease despite the apparent herd immunity.

Herd effect also relies on the assumption that the development of a disease in an individual can only occur, after being infected with the disease agent from somebody that has symptoms of the actual disease, and therefore assumes that you cannot get the disease agent from asymptomatic carriers, i.e. from people with the microbes that have no symptoms of illness.

> *Meningococcal bacteria are carried in many of us, they are conceivably passed around from host to host but will only cause disease when a patient becomes susceptible, even from a fairly orthodox point of view, carrying microbes and having disease are two separate things.*

Given that asymptomatic carriage is a reality, then the vaccine would not only have to create immunity but would have to physically eliminate the microbe from the entire person, the community and consequently from the world. However, being immune to illness does not mean the body doesn't harbour a potential pathogen in other appropriate areas of the body, even if vaccines could create immunity, vaccines have never been shown to eliminate pathogens entirely from the body.

If the assumptions of herd immunity are correct then disease could not start in highly vaccinated populations above the herd immunity threshold.

> *"Many outbreaks (measles) have occurred among school-aged children in schools with vaccination levels above 98%. These outbreaks have occurred in all parts of the country."*

> The Morbidity and Mortality Weekly Report'
> (MMWR) CDC 13/01/89-38(1); 11-14

Some vaccines, for example the vaccine for diphtheria toxin, could in theory aid the blood immune response to the toxin from the bacteria but does not stop the bacteria proliferating on the mucus membranes or skin of the body therefore has no chance of creating a herd effect.

"...Immunization with diphtheria toxoid is protective only against the phage-mediated toxin and not against infection by the C. diphtheriae organism... Outbreaks in communities with up to 94 per cent immunization levels have been reported. Therefore, some authors have challenged whether "herd immunity" is applicable to diphtheria."

R.T. Chen, M.D. et al.
American Journal of Public Health, Dec 1985, Vol 75, No.12

But the main assumption underpinning herd immunity from the point of view of vaccination is of course that the vaccine affects the human body in the same way as natural immunity i.e. that it works, and that it works to a very high degree, given that many thresholds are upwards of 90%. For example assuming all the calculations and assumptions are correct to calculate this theoretical threshold, if you need a herd immunity of 90% the vaccine would have to have an efficacy of greater than 90% or the target could never be reached. A vaccine less than 90% effective could not create 90% population immunity even if you vaccinated 100% of the population. Whether the vaccine works or not is of course the whole debate and at best it has <u>never</u> been shown to operate in the same way as natural immunity, hence the need for repeat booster shots of vaccines as vaccinated individuals continue to succumb to the vaccinated disease, which is of course unlike natural immunity.

Therefore the idea that we need a certain percentage uptake of vaccine to create the desired threshold of 'herd immunity' in order to safeguard everyone, even those not vaccinated, through the 'herd effect' and thus eliminate the disease from the world, is a mathematical *theory* taken from *assumptions* about the natural decline in diseases that is then superimposed on vaccine theory. The mathematical equations that describe the incidence of disease in populations are very complex and are entirely different for different illnesses; they are approximate and hypothetical mathematical descriptions of the relationships between individuals and the conditions that give rise to illness, and they leave out some of the most important factors pertaining to illness in the real world.

Regarding the actual percentage vaccine uptake required in the population, and the required re-vaccination rate, to eradicate an illness, this has of course different estimates according to the different mathematical models used and also varies from illness to illness, but more significantly it has **never** been demonstrated in practice for any vaccinated disease.

The basic assumption that you can eliminate disease from the world, by sufficient people being immune, requires that these microbes can only exist when we have the disease and that they cannot exist if we are immune. However, it is common knowledge that individuals harbour microbes and do not have disease, therefore even if vaccines could reduce illness, they have never been shown to totally rid the body of the germ. Herd immunity and the eradication of disease, from the point of view of the vaccine induced herd effect, is a flawed hypothesis.

5.3 Smallpox

The only illness said to have been eradicated by vaccination is smallpox (although cases are still said to exist under a different classification) and interestingly the eradication is supposed to have occurred worldwide when in fact vaccine uptake rates were nothing like what they were supposed to be in order to achieve herd immunity.

> *"The disappearance of smallpox from many regions despite the continued presence of large numbers of unvaccinated susceptibles was evident from the historical record (as had been noted by Farr more than a century ago)."*

> Paul E.M. Fine Epidemiologic Reviews 1993
> Johns Hopkins University, Vol. 15, No. 2

More importantly it was the only mass vaccinated illness before the 1900's and the only illness to <u>increase</u> in death rate after the use of the vaccine, whilst all other illnesses were in decline without the use of vaccines. The symptoms of smallpox are still evident according to the World Health Organisation, only now the clinically identical illnesses are classified by different names for example 'monkey pox'. The real biochemical proof of eradication is said to be due to the fact that the vaccine virus is not found in the natural world. Given that the vaccine viral components have been so dramatically changed over time in the ongoing production of vaccines, it is highly probable that no naturally occurring virus or similar DNA thought to be from the virus looks anything like the supposed smallpox components in the vaccine. The virus hasn't been eradicated, it's just that vaccine manufacturers have produced a vaccine virus that cannot be found in the natural world.

From the vaccine promoters point of reference obviously the more people vaccinated the better, however there is no verifiable percentage uptake that leads to the elimination of the disease, this is a complete mathematical hypothesis unproven with regard to any vaccine, and in any disease situation. If vaccines work, then the 'vaccinated' are protected, and they need not worry about those that choose to not vaccinate. The fact that vaccines cannot be given to sick people, the very people that need intervention to increase their immune function shows the potential problems with vaccines, problems that are not evident from any other natural immune enhancing intervention. Alternative and natural therapeutics, unlike vaccines, are actually designed for the sick.

CHAPTER SIX

6 Do vaccine promoters really understand the causes of disease?

"When you trust in yourself you trust in the wisdom that created you"

Dr Wayne Dyer
Author and International Speaker on Self development

The human body responds intelligently to changes in the external environment in ways that allow the internal cellular surroundings to remain fairly constant, this is vital because the functioning of the body can only occur within a certain range of conditions.

When these reactions are perceived to be uncomfortable, are they any less intelligent?

If we are able to understand the purpose of our reactions, even during symptoms of disease, would this change our perspective and therefore our ability to treat disease?

6.1 The human body - Intelligent by design

All life forms have mechanisms that are capable of responding to changes in temperature, humidity, nutritional levels, oxygen, carbon dioxide, acidity, light, perceived danger and so on, and of course none more so than the sophisticated physiology of the human being. If, for example, the external environment gets colder, our internal system heats up to compensate, if we have insufficient intake of water then the kidneys retain more water, etc. This process of internal balancing is called homeostasis and in fact, the body can only remain alive whilst these coordinated responses are working.

6.1.1 Toxic waste - a fact of life

However, not only are there external influences on the body that we have to adapt to, but there are also those created by our own internal metabolism. 'Metabolism' is a word to describe the overall chemical reactions of the human body - taking in food substances to be oxidised (burnt) in the presence of oxygen, thereby releasing energy, and the incorporation of these food substances to renew and create the structures of the human body. The accompanying accumulation of by-products is generally toxic and consequently these waste products need to be eliminated, the production of this waste, effectively toxins, occurs even if we could conceivably ingest no toxins at all, therefore toxin elimination is something the body is extremely efficient at doing, it has to be, in order to stay alive.

When dealing with health and illness the issue of toxicity within the body is paramount. A toxin is any substance that can adversely affect the function of your cells and there are many kinds of toxins affecting different cells in a variety of ways. Therefore because our normal metabolism produces toxins, we have many mechanisms in place to eliminate these potentially harmful substances, and sometimes if these toxins are particularly dangerous they will have to go through a chemical process of deactivation, often in the liver, before they are eliminated from the body.

The following processes as well as performing other functions, also serve as the main mechanisms of elimination.

      a.   Perspiration - Skin
      b.   Respiration - Lungs
      c.   Urination - Kidneys
      d.   Defaecation - Bowels

6.1.2 Assembling the parts - an introduction to holism

"Science is built up of facts, as a house is built of stones; but an accumulation of facts is no more a science than a heap of stones is a house."

Henri Poincaré, Science and Hypothesis, 1905

For the purposes of toxicity and elimination, the body can be described as having an inside and outside. The inside, being separated from the outside, by a physical membrane, our 'skin'. Pierce the skin and you will expose our internal systems, blood, tissues etc to the external environment.

Our skin covers the entire body, and at the mouth, the skin continues into the cavity of the digestive system, via the lips, maintaining this barrier into our digestive tract. The skin, lining the mouth, is different from our external skin; in the mouth it is a mucous membrane, but nevertheless it is a skin continuous with your outer skin covering the body. This membrane continues through the length of our digestive tract through the throat, stomach, small intestine and large intestine until it reaches the anus, whereupon it forms a continuous membrane with our skin once again. It is as though the digestive tract from mouth to anus forms a continuous tube through the body, much like the whole though a doughnut.

It is important to have a general understanding of the inside and outside of the body from the perspective of your skin and mucous membrane. Although the body can be divided into parts, a whole body perspective of 'in and out' allows us to appreciate the purpose of various symptoms in disease and the priorities of the body in terms of development, protection and ultimately survival.

Diagrammatical representation:
Digestive tract running through the body

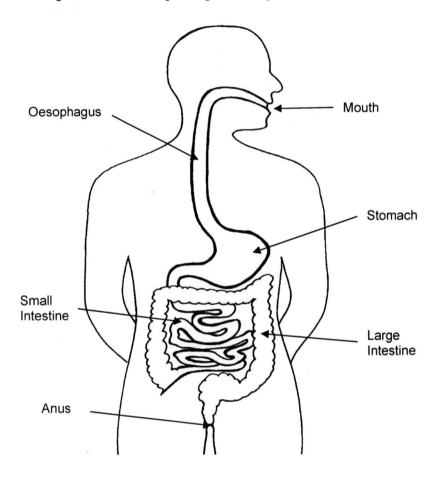

Therefore anything within the cavity of your mouth can still be considered to be outside of your body, i.e. it is not until a substance passes across this membrane that it is actually internalised. Consequently anything in your stomach and intestines can be considered to be outside of your body until it passes across the membrane lining the stomach and intestine. If you were to swallow something relatively small and indigestible like a glass marble, this would pass right through your digestive tract: mouth, throat, stomach, small intestine and large intestine and be passed out through your anus and at no time would it have been internalised into your body.

This is the way we shall consider inside and outside of the body for the purposes of this part of our discussion. A similar situation can be said to exist for other parts of the body also, the lungs, ear, nose and throat also bladder and kidneys.

Diagrammatical representation
Respiratory tract and Urinary tract running into the body

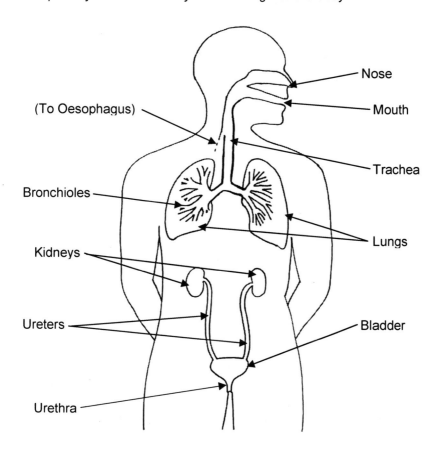

Now these structures (lungs and kidneys) do not have tubes that pass right through our bodies like the digestive system, but generally consist of tubes that are blocked off at their ends that also separate the internal tissues by a membrane that is once again continuous with the outer skin.

In the elimination of toxins, the waste products of our metabolism are usually eliminated into these spaces: The large intestine for defaecation, the kidneys and bladder for urination, the skin in perspiration and the lungs during respiration, whereupon they are then expelled completely from the body.

This toxin elimination is a very important part of our immune function and the presence of the **membrane** is an important structure involved in these processes. There are elements present on these membranes that are important for the functioning of the membrane: cilia (fine hairs), bacteria and viruses, mucus and other secretions, acid or alkali solutions, enzymes, immune chemicals, non-specific antibodies (immunoglobulins) and white blood cells.

6.1.3 Ingestion of toxins

As well as the normal production of toxins from our metabolism, we also know that toxins can be ingested into the body, for example through our digestive system from food and drink, through our lungs via air pollution and smoking, and through our skin from cosmetics, pollutants in washing water and other elements in contact with the skin. All of which will need to be eliminated as described above.

6.2 Symptoms - Function or Mal-Function?

> *"Disease is not a meaningless "error" of nature or biology but a special program created by nature over millions of years of evolution to allow organisms to override everyday functioning and to deal with particular emergency situations; they are wonderful programs and, if understood*

correctly, provide the individual and the group with a way to deal with "out of the ordinary" circumstances".

Dr Ryke Geerd Hamer

We know that certain factors can lead to an accumulation of excess toxins in these external body spaces, digestive tract, upper ear, nose and throat, lungs, bladder, etc:

1. Sudden or gradual increase of ingested toxins: -
    From our diet, drug habits, environmental pollution etc.
2. Reduced capacity of organs to eliminate: -
    Due to physical, mental or emotional stress
3. Nutritional deficiencies: -
    Contribute to the inability of the body to carry out basic eliminatory functions.
4. Direct suppression of our elimination responses: -
    From the use of antiperspirants etc.

If we are able to eliminate these toxins as fast as they accumulate then our normal function of perspiration, respiration, urination and defaecation is sufficient to eliminate toxicity.

If however our normal functions were unable to eliminate toxins fast enough then the accumulation of toxins would provoke an increased elimination response from your body:

> ➤ Vomiting and diarrhoea.
> ➤ Respiratory mucus with coughing, sneezing and nasal discharge.
> ➤ Pimples that discharge, increased sweating and urination, with increased concentration and odour.

The function of these responses at this stage would be to increase toxin elimination over and above the normal physiological responses of perspiration, respiration, urination and defaecation: These increased responses are now associated with feelings of discomfort, we now experience **symptoms** of 'dis-ease'. There may be some debate as to when you decide some reactions are symptoms, for example profuse sweating in extreme heat or physical activity will not be considered a symptom of illness because the reaction is not disproportionate to the activity of the person. Diarrhoea, vomiting, coughing and sneezing will, more often than not, be considered symptomatic of illness unless there is an immediate and benign cause.

Generally before the onset of symptoms you would have been able to eliminate all toxins through your **normal 'function'**, and therefore with no discomfort (perspiration − skin, respiration − lungs, urination − kidneys, defaecation - bowels) but at the stage of an excessive build up of toxicity, an increased response is necessary, therefore **'symptoms'** are experienced; sweating and urination with increased odour and concentration, vomiting, diarrhoea, respiratory mucus/cough/sneeze etc. With the increased toxins within these spaces of the body the altered toxic conditions now encourage other microbes to multiply which brings us once again to the question of the role of microbes in disease. These microbes proliferate as a result of the underlying condition and are therefore not the primary cause, they may help to clean up the environment and return the body to normal conditions, but with their concomitant waste they may however also add something to the toxicity.

6.3 Microbes and their association with toxicity

6.3.1 Koch's Postulates

In 1890 the German physician and bacteriologist Robert Koch set out his celebrated criteria for judging whether a given bacteria is the cause of a given disease. These criteria are taught to this day and are used by scientists to help them decide whether a given bacteria can be defined as being responsible for a particular disease. Koch's criteria brought some much-needed scientific clarity to what was then a very confused field.

Koch's postulates are as follows:

> ➢ The bacteria must be present in every case of the disease.
> ➢ The bacteria must be isolated from the host with the disease and grown in pure culture.
> ➢ The specific disease must be reproduced when a pure culture of the bacteria is inoculated into a healthy susceptible host.
> ➢ The bacteria must be recoverable from the experimentally infected host.

However, Koch's postulates have their limitations and so may not always be the last word. They may not hold if:

> ➢ The particular bacteria cannot be "grown in pure culture" in the laboratory.
> ➢ There is no animal 'model' of infection that accurately mimics the human illness in which to carry out experiments.
> ➢ The bacteria can only cause disease when introduced into the body in ways that do not naturally occur.

In addition a harmless bacterium may cause disease if:

> ➢ It gains access to deep tissues via trauma, bites, injections, surgery, etc.
> ➢ It is present in an immuno-compromised patient.

And even in bacteria that appear to be demonstrably pathogenic (associated with disease), in fact not all people infected by the bacteria develop disease, sub-clinical infection is usually **more common** than clinically obvious infection, i.e. although many individuals have the bacteria **most show no symptoms of disease**.

Hib, Meningococcal and E.coli bacteria are all supposed to cause meningitis yet most of us have all these bacteria within our systems all the time with no symptoms of illness. Evidence of viruses; HPV, HIV, herpes and polio though found in huge proportions of the population, yet again for the vast majority they are associated with no symptoms of disease.

Despite such limitations, Koch's postulates are still used as a benchmark in judging whether there is a correlation between a bacteria (or any other type of microorganism) and a clinical disease. However, until further investigations are carried out, this will only tell us which microbes are present at the time of certain diseases but cannot tell us as yet whether they 'caused' the condition or are the 'result' of the condition. For example we will always find flies around the cow dung deposited in the grazing fields of cows but flies are clearly not responsible for depositing them there, flies are associated with cow dung in cow fields though not causative, consequently they are part of the effect but not the cause.

6.4 Bacteria - a necessary fact of life

Of the billions of microbes within the human body a large percentage of them occupy the spaces in contact with your mucous membranes and external skin, most appear to be external to your body fluids. Therefore although these elements are in the digestive, urinary and respiratory tracts they are essentially, as previously defined, **<u>outside of the body</u>**.

If you imagine the total number of cells in your entire body (estimated at around 50,000,000,000,000) then the number of **microbes** within the human body would be 10 times greater than the number of your own cells, of which **90% are in the digestive tract**. (The Lancet Vol. 360, Feb 08, 2003)

The microbes in the digestive tract are collectively known as the gut flora, and have many functions:

> ➤ Resist colonization of other bacteria and fungus from our normal environment.

> ➤ Digestion of residues from the upper intestines that we are unable to digest with our own enzymes.
> ➤ Salvage of energy by producing short chain fatty acids for use by the body.
> ➤ Production of vitamins for the body
> ➤ Aid mineral absorption.
> ➤ Stimulate normal growth of intestinal cells (laboratory studies show they can also reverse cancer growth)

The gut microbes represent the larger fraction of our microbial friends but there are of course more on the membranes of other tissues; the lungs, ears, nose, throat, genitourinary tracts and our skin. It is also known that these microbes can change their form, under toxic conditions and may produce additional bacterial toxic waste, in an already toxic environment. Bacteria are known to decompose dead tissue but do not 'attack' living tissue, as is often implied by our concept of disease-causing germs. We live in a symbiotic relationship with our microbes; part of a necessary ecosystem of the normal functioning healthy body.

6.4.1 Bacteria and the immune system in partnership

Recent research published in Public Library of Science (PLoS) Pathogens 22/07/2005, has also shown that bacteria not only regulate the numbers of other microbes by competing for space and resources but are able reduce opposing numbers by **working with the immune cells of the human body**. Literally calling in white blood cells (in this instance the white blood cells are neutrophils) to eradicate competing bacteria, researchers at the University Of Pennsylvania School Of Medicine studying two strains of bacteria normally present in the upper respiratory tract, found that one strain H. influenzae would attract white blood cells to kill off its rival S. pneumoniae.

> *"The results of this study show that recognition of microbial products from one species may activate inflammatory responses that promote the clearance of another competing*

*species. This study also demonstrates how **manipulations such as antibiotics or vaccines**, which are meant to diminish the presence of a single pathogen, may inadvertently alter the competitive interactions of complex microbial communities."*

The results are being used to explain the side-effects of the pneumonia vaccine that is resulting in more middle ear infections.

So we have evidence from up to date microbiological studies demonstrating how attempts to eliminate one type of bacteria causes imbalances in the body and increased diseases, facts that appear to be unknown to vaccine producers. This also throws into question our assumptions as to the causes of disease, the presence of bacteria in disease may also be caused by imbalances and not just by marauding bacteria that we need to kill.

6.4.2 Microbes changing form

Also as previously mentioned there are the many scientists since the 1900s; Dr Gunther Enderlein; Dr Rife, Dr Gaston Naessens, Dr Wilhelm Reich that have observed and demonstrated the ability of microbes to change form dramatically; changing into various types of bacteria and to fungal colonies and even creating viral particles.

Scientists working with live blood samples, using what is called 'darkfield' or 'dark phase' microscopy, are able to observe microbes changing into these different forms according to the nature of their environment; the more acidic, the less oxygenated and the more polluted the bodily fluid, the more we find associated microbes. As acidity and toxicity levels increase and oxygen concentrations decrease these microbes grow larger and accumulate protein reserves as an adaptation to their environment and practitioners are able to remedy diseases by addressing the conditions that create internal toxicity.

This ability of microbes to exhibit such extreme morphological change is called 'pleomorphism' and has historically been rejected by the orthodox medical establishment, although conventional scientists have more recently recognised many instances of pleomorphism. In addition, as published in the Journal of Clinical Microbiology, August 16 2002, conventional microbiological methods, have demonstrated the existence of populations of pleomorphic bacteria in healthy human blood, the internal fluid of the body that was always thought to be sterile in healthy individuals.

6.4.3 Dr Ryke Geerd Hamer

Additionally in the resolution of cancer tumours, many researchers have found that they often contain bacteria, and different tumours are consistently associated with different types of bacteria. Dr Ryke Geerd Hamer has an exceptionally high success rate with his cancer therapy; the public prosecutor's office of Wiener Neustadt examined 6500 patient cases from Burgau, who were considered incurable by traditional medical standards. Surprisingly, over 90% of these patients had survived, i.e. over 6000 using the methods of Dr Hamer. He has noted the presence of bacteria in tumour cells that have the function of destroying and digesting the tumour as an integral part of the healing response to cancer.

Dr Hamer's observations are being used by large numbers of practitioners; he has also demonstrated that significant emotional traumas will be interpreted by the patient in a way that reflects their own specific sensitivities and fears. He has distinguished four main types of emotional susceptibilities; separation trauma, fear of survival, fear of attack and self-devaluation, each will impact on a specific part of the body and will nave a corresponding impact in the brain as seen with an MRI scan. The brain part affected will be reflective of the developmental tissue layer in embryology and will therefore correspond exactly to the appropriate part of the body. Thereby body-part, brain and emotion are exactly correlated and the role of the microbe is not seen as an indiscriminate agent, attacking the body, but an integral part of its healing mechanism in the breakdown of specific diseased tissue.

These facts are however still largely ignored by the present orthodoxy in terms of their practical approach to treating disease, mainly because they appear to undermine their own perspective and approach to treating illness. Orthodox interpretations tend to think of microbes as static elements unable to change form, known as monomorphism, and that pathogenic microbes are either present or not and that healthy human blood is sterile and therefore free of microbes. Consequently the way to deal with illness and the associated microbes, is simply to kill them.

There are of course major consequences to accepting the existence of microbes in healthy human blood and the phenomena of pleomorphism:

- ➢ Firstly the nature of the 'terrain' i.e. the body fluids, determines the nature and amount of microbe present, therefore it is much more imperative to address the nature of the terrain as determined by, diet, toxins, lifestyle, etc. as opposed to merely killing microbes.

- ➢ Secondly according to the research of dark field microscopists, many of these microbes already exist within the blood, therefore not only do we have a widely accepted source of good bacteria and others associated with disease on our skin and mucous membranes (i.e. on the outside spaces of the body), the implication is that they can potentially exist on the inside, in places of the body that we previously thought were 'sterile', (i.e. containing no microbes at all – in particular bacteria).

- ➢ These bacteria exist in symbiotic balance with each other and in close relationship to the immune system; killing off some microbes will have wider implications, unintentionally compromising others and the functioning of the immune system.

> ➢ Thirdly, these microbes, like those that have been found in cancer tumours, are thought to have the ability to digest surrounding toxins, and dead tissue and thereby are an **aid to immune function** rather than the primary cause of disease.

6.5 Antibiotics in principle

With the proliferation of bacteria in diseased patients, antimicrobials may help to destroy microbes and thus slow down the cleanup process, creating some time for the human body to address toxic and microbial imbalances, they could certainly create some respite from microbial toxins. They may also be useful, especially as a last resort, when innate healing systems appear to be overloaded and in cases where microbes have infected the internal systems from the skin and mucous membranes from injuries and immune damage. But there are some potential problems with the use of antimicrobials that need to be factored in when designing protocols for managing disease.

Firstly, it is recognised within orthodox medicine that the elimination of bacteria by the use of antibiotics as a first resort does not allow the immune system to develop its own natural ability to deal with such imbalances.

Secondly, many of the bacteria that are important for health are also destroyed and this upsets the balance of healthy bacteria within the body and can predispose the patient to other opportunistic infections from bacteria or fungus associated with illness. Fungal symptoms of thrush are a common consequence of antibiotic treatment.

This effect can have even more severe consequences in new born children. In the first days of life babies develop a tolerance to appropriate populations of beneficial bacteria, however, the use of antibiotics at this stage can increase the likelihood of microbes associated with illness colonising their digestive tracts on a more permanent basis, not just for the period whilst taking antibiotics. It has been demonstrated that such children can find it very difficult to maintain healthy populations of beneficial bacteria right into adulthood and are predisposed to digestive disturbances, inflammatory conditions, systemic fungal conditions, blood toxicity, neurological problems, allergies, colon cancer and whole host of related illnesses.

Thirdly, the microbial response to 'disease' rather than being the cause may in fact be part of the curative response and therefore the body's method of utilising microbes to digest dead tissue and toxins, killing these microbes will therefore have a detrimental effect on the patient.

Fourthly, the antibiotic itself is a poisonous chemical that has to be detoxified and then eliminated from the body, this would then actually add to the problem if in fact we are already struggling with an overburdened immune system and increased toxic load.

In addition, if the predisposing factors of diet or toxic build-up from other sources are not addressed, then killing the pathogenic bacteria would only make way for the production of more pathogenic bacteria, produced from the vast pool of existing bacteria within the system.

If antibiotics have been used, then the least resistant strains are killed first, leaving a certain number of the most resistant strains surviving. This is why we are asked to finish a course of antibiotics; to kill off all the last remaining, and most resistant strains. However, this is an empty rhetoric; there will <u>always</u> be some survivors and so long as the predisposing factors are not dealt with, then these microbes along with any predecessors to pathogenic bacteria will then create the new dominant forms of bacteria.

These forms will be resistant to the initial antibiotic and so a new antibiotic will be needed. This cycle of administering antibiotics and leaving the most resistant strains left can continue until the predominant bacteria surviving are resistant to all the known forms of antibiotic and we would have created the 'superbug'.

This so-called super-bug is no more capable of creating symptoms of illness than any other bug, it just happens to be resistant to our antibiotics. If the predisposing factors are not addressed then these bacteria will dominate and proliferate contributing to the consequences of disease. Because many holistic practitioners do not give antibiotics and prefer instead to address the conditions that cause and maintain these microbes, then illnesses associated with so-called super-bugs can be treated just as easily as any other condition involving other microbes.

The superbug is <u>not</u> a consequence of unclean hospitals and treatment centres, they may be spread because of poor cleanliness but they are formed by the overuse of antibiotics and in fact they tend to be most common in the cleanest parts of the hospital; intensive care units, surgical wards and operating theatres. They are a direct consequence of antibiotic treatment with the concomitant disregard of the causative factors of the illness.

It is possible that after the use of antibiotics, the human body can redress the toxic imbalance; eliminating toxins through vomiting, diarrhoea, mucus discharge, fasting through natural loss of appetite, bed rest, inflammatory responses etc. Antibiotics can slow this down and so appear to give you time, and may be useful as a last resort, however, unless the underlying toxicity issues have been addressed then the antibiotic is ultimately useless, microbes will continue to grow and prolonged use of antibiotics may eventually create more problems than they solve.

6.6 The role of viruses in disease.

Having made the assumption that inflammatory reactions, the formation of rashes and the production of mucus and other discharges, were the definitive signs of 'infection', scientists then discovered that exactly those symptoms could be produced without bacteria.

Before modern scientific techniques were able to isolate, characterise and photograph minute particles, it was initially inferred that these illnesses were caused by microscopic elements called viruses, which eventually lead to the search and characterisation for these new pathogens. These viruses quickly became the new physiological enemy, the definitive bio-terrorist, and many so-called infectious illnesses were defined by the specific virus that were thought to be the cause of the illness; measles, rubella, chickenpox, AIDS, polio, etc.

However the issue of viral causation in disease is far from clear; remember that Koch defined the basic criteria by which scientists could determine whether an illness could be defined as being caused by a microbe (mainly for bacteria and protozoa single-cell organisms).

> The bacteria must be present in every case of the disease.
> The bacteria must be isolated from the host with the disease and grown in pure culture.
> The specific disease must be reproduced when a pure culture of the bacteria is inoculated into a healthy susceptible host.

These Koch's Postulates were however redefined in 1937 and 1982 in an attempt to accommodate the new diseases that were thought to be caused by viruses.

Redefined because, many viruses could easily exist in humans that do not cause disease; many could not be isolated and identified in cases of disease; many could not cause illness through skin contact, breathed in or ingested through the digestive tract but only if injected in large quantities directly into the body, which of course is not the method by which most of these illnesses are contracted.

6.6.1 What are viruses?

Viruses are effectively small packets of genes, chemically composed of DNA or RNA. Genes are the information that the cell uses to reproduce exact copies of itself and they also provide a blue-print for the production of proteins that determine the structure and function of each cell.

6.6.2 Viruses are not alive

A virus is a very small amount of this genetic material covered in a protective coat, viruses are much smaller than bacteria and although we talk of 'live vaccines' implying the virus is still alive, viruses themselves are not living things. 'Live' from the point of view of vaccine manufacturers really means 'not destroyed' or 'not chemically annihilated' or not a genetically engineered chemical copy.

A virus contains **only** genetic information and has no other elements capable of digesting, eliminating, reproducing, moving, etc. It can carry out **none** of the functions requisite for life; a virus is basically a sophisticated chemical. However, the genetic information from the virus can be taken in by a host cell and in some instances they can be reproduced by that host cell producing more viral copies. There are in fact many kinds of viruses in almost all forms of life; plants, animals and bacteria.

The controversy lies in the significance of viruses in disease and therefore the **viral disease theory**. As with other microbes, we have been told that:

The virus is the cause of many viral illnesses and can only infect from outside of the host or cell. Once within the host cell, the host reproduces the virus in great number, very rapidly, (the virus is not capable of doing this on its own), and consequently the host cell dies, bursts open and releases many more viruses into the tissue of the body, whereupon they are able to infect more cells. These infected cells are then hijacked to reproduce more viruses in the same manner as before, thereby causing symptoms of disease and in severe cases the eventual death of the host.

However, there are considerable problems with this theory, problems that in many ways mirror the situation with bacteria.

> Most viruses that infect bacteria, plants, and animals (including humans) do not cause disease. In fact, scientists have studied viruses at length and have found those that infect bacteria may be helpful, in that they rapidly transfer genetic information from one bacterium to another. Viruses of plants and animals may convey genetic information among similar species, aiding the survival of their hosts in hostile environments.

> **Encyclopedia Britannica, Macropaedia (1990) p507:**
> **Recited in "Images of Polio" – by Jim West**

> This method of acquiring genes is not in doubt. Bacteria as well as higher animal cells including humans are known to acquire viral genes, and the phenomenon is not rare. Endogenous viruses and viral elements have been found in all vertebrates investigated. As a general rule, the number of groups of viral sequences found within a given vertebrate species is proportional to the effort spent searching that species, i.e. whenever we look we find them and the more we look the more we find.

> The supposed AIDS virus, HIV, is said to be responsible for the immune breakdown of a patient with symptoms of AIDS, by the insertion of viral genetic information into the genes of patient's T-cells. It is very difficult to conceive how such a small amount of nucleic acid that is supposed to be found in only 1% of T-cells can account for the range of pathology seen in AIDS. Recently it has become known that approximately 3,000 times that amount of viral DNA already exists in normal cells. (Eleni Papadopulos-Eleopulos, in Continuum, Autumn 1997). The connection between AIDS and HIV is extremely controversial many of the original researchers do not even accept that the HIV is responsible for AIDS.

➤ Scientists have also demonstrated the ability of **cells** to **produce viruses** when under threat from external poisons and radiation, it is known as the SOS response in bacteria. This is in fact part of the reaction to poisons that is used to find out how toxic a chemical is, it is a standard chemical test used in the pharmaceutical industry and agrochemical industry to assess the toxicity of additives, drugs and insecticides called the 'Ames' test. The production of viruses under such circumstances could be:

◊ A method of informing or warning other cells of the danger
◊ Instructing other cells how to affect the required response to the trauma, just as genetic resistance to antibiotics can be transferred to other bacteria in this manner.
◊ The packaging of the DNA codes as with other cell components to be recycled and used by other cells.

➤ Therefore, rather than the cause of cell breakdown, we know that viruses are caused by the poisoning of cells, the cell effectively breaks up and packages tiny amounts of its genetic material in protective membranes, these are in fact viruses. A poisoned cell effectively produces viruses, therefore it is very likely that the reason why so much viral DNA/RNA is found in normal cellular DNA is because that is where the viral DNA actually came from, viruses are in fact broken up pieces of our own cellular DNA.

➤ We also know that viruses transfer useful genetic information from cell to cell and to other individuals in <u>healthy</u> cells, yet surprisingly we have **never** been able to show a virus infecting a host cell from the outside to create a diseased cell. In the decades of viral research using electron microscopes able to detect small particles such as viruses, we have never been able to show what is known as 'infectosomes' in diseased cells, i.e. viruses being incorporated in the membrane of a host cell transferring genetic information into the cell causing its disease and destruction.

> All examples of supposed viral elements in disease seem to corroborate the fact that these elements are caused by poisoning cells first and they are in fact the breakdown products of the cell. Dying cells will often breakdown internally, packaging up its molecular components in membrane bound portions. In programmed cell death this process is called apoptosis. The transfer of these supposed viruses to other cells although they can be incorporated in healthy cells does not subsequently create disease in those cells.

> Additionally, because the normal products of cells follow a line of activity from genes in the nucleus to outside of the nucleus, scientists naturally assumed that any 'back-flow' was pathological. There was an assumption that activity should not flow back into the nucleus affecting the genes. This 'Reverse Transcription' as it is called, was deemed pathology, a mal-function, a cause of disease, and was assumed to be caused by a virus that was changing the patients DNA or inserting its own viral DNA in the patient. However we have since learnt that this activity often occurs when the cell is carrying out normal DNA repair, it is more likely to be occurring as a result of disease rather than causing a disease.

In fact many illnesses that are diagnosed as viral have never had a positive identification of such; it is usually a diagnosis by default, if nothing else can be found then it's probably viral.

Expensive lab tests involve characterising the DNA of assumed viruses; this is rarely performed on patients that are ill. Very occasionally a clinical test for the antibodies to a virus is used which infers the presence of a virus but again this is subject to interpretation. There isn't a reliable clinical test for the viruses themselves, so the actual virus is not tested for, just the presence of antibodies to the virus. It is therefore highly probable that viruses may be present but with undetectable levels of antibody to them. As such, not only are there inherent problems in ascertaining whether a virus is the cause of an illness, but additional problems in ascertaining whether a virus is actually there or not and if it is present, whether it has 'infected' the host or always been there.

The HIV test is in fact a test for an antibody to a protein that has been assumed to be from the virus, but the virus has <u>never been isolated</u>. In addition most people will in fact test positive for the presence of this antibody, but there has been an agreed concentration of antibody that suddenly defines whether you are HIV positive or not. Below that concentration you are considered negative; above that you are considered positive, therefore this does <u>not</u> state that someone who is HIV positive has the antibody and someone who is HIV negative does not. Those testing negative could and often do have lower levels of these antibodies.

Dr Stefan Lanka a German research scientist having studied molecular biology and ecology started viral research in 1986. Then as the public became aware of AIDS and its connection with a virus (HIV), he was automatically considered an expert on AIDS. However when checking the literature of previous research on AIDS he found that scientists were not providing proof of a virus. Dr Lanka was deeply shocked but wanted to be sure...

"Well, I'm not experienced enough. I have overlooked something. On the other side, those people are absolutely sure. Then I was afraid that speaking about this with my friends, or even my family, they would think is absolutely mad and crazy. So for a long time I studied virology, from the end to the beginning, from the beginning to the end, to be absolutely sure that there was no such thing as HIV. And it was easy for me to be sure about this because I realized that the whole group of viruses to which HIV is said to belong, the retroviruses -- as well as other viruses which are claimed to be very dangerous -- in fact do not exist at all."...

"For almost one year we have been asking authorities, politicians and medical institutes after the scientific evidence for the existence of such viruses that are said to cause disease and therefore require "immunization". After almost one year we have not received even one concrete answer which provides evidence for the existence of those "vaccination viruses". The conclusion is inevitable that our children are still vaccinated on the basis of scientific standards of the 18th and 19th century. In the 19th century Robert Koch demanded in his generally accepted postulates evidence of the virus in order to prove infection; at Koch's time this evidence couldn't be achieved directly by visualization and characterization of the viruses, because adequate technology wasn't available at that time. Methods of modern medicine have profoundly changed over the past 60 years, in particular by the invention of the electron microscope. And still all these viruses we get immunized against have never been re-examined using this technology?"...

Regarding the available photographic proof of viruses studied by Dr Lanka:

"All these photos have in common that they, (the authors), can't claim that they present a virus, as long as they do not also provide the original publications which describe how and what from the virus has been isolated. Such original publications are cited **nowhere**. Indeed, in the entire scientific literature there's not even one publication, where "viruses in the disease" the fulfillment of Koch's first postulate is even claimed. That means that there is no proof that from humans with certain diseases the viruses - which are held responsible for these diseases - have been isolated. Nevertheless, this is precisely what they publicly claim."

www.klein-klein-aktion.de

The role of microbes as causative agents of disease is indeed sketchy; in fact techniques in most of the alternative therapies have focused on detoxification, immune building, adding friendly bacteria and working with the elimination procedures of the body, etc. None of which have ever required a positive identification of a microbe that has needed to be killed.

Summary

Let us now be clear about these issues, bacteria and fungus are living micro-organisms (unlike viruses), what is in question is their role in the 'causation' of disease, and more particularly infectious disease. Bacteria and fungus can be utilised by the body to digest toxins even though this process of digestion can produce other toxic byproducts some of which can also cause symptoms, the disease causation would have been the initial toxicity and cellular breakdown. As such you cannot catch these diseases from someone else unless your cellular environment is the same as the next person, in which case you are reacting to your circumstances, eliminating toxins, and thereby cultivating microbes, you do not have a disease that was caused by catching a microbe.

Bacteria and fungus can also contaminate the body from an external source if for example you were to ingest decayed and contaminated food these germs would add to your toxicity; as such we have an issue of food/water poisoning, not an infectious disease, even if you could irradiate and kill microbes from such contaminated food, the food quality itself would still cause illness because it is no longer nutritious but poisonous.

Additionally, an injury to one part of our body can allow microbes to enter and therefore contaminate other parts of our body that are ordinarily relatively microbe free, thus causing symptoms of disease, again this is a special case caused by injury and not an infectious disease.

Viruses on the other hand are not living microbes, they have not been demonstrated as the cause of disease, they are mostly present in stable relationships with certain host cells and have only been isolated, characterised and electron-micrographed (i.e. photographed) in primitive cells. Rather than a demonstrable cause of disease, viruses have been verified as being caused by the poisoning of cells and have never been found to infect cells in disease tissue, furthermore none have ever been characterised by the techniques currently available in modern virology. Their presence is by inference by indirect supposition, but what is particularly damning is that the technology to isolate, characterise and electron micrograph viruses is in fact now readily available but has so far not been able to demonstrate the presence or causation of viruses in disease tissue.

The viral story is quite an incredible tale going back to the days of Edward Jenner and the imagined smallpox virus to the present day, with virus classifications apparently based on membrane proteins, enzymes and genetic material. But here the perspective of virologist Stefan Lanka is quite instructive, he shows how in fact the viral disease theories are based on belief systems creating hypothesis, leading to assumption and more supposition, inferred from very limited biological experiments, none of which has been verified using the techniques we now have available in modern science.

> *"If ever a virus coming from a specific body or a body fluid, for instance from birds, has been proven, then any average scientist can verify, in any average laboratory, within a day, whether this virus is present in for instance a dead animal. This has however never occurred, and on the contrary, indirect test methods which tell absolutely nothing are being used."*
>
> Stefan Lanka

6.7 How do they know that viruses are present in disease?

6.7.1 Viral anti-bodies

In trying to assess if a given virus is present scientists test the body for antibodies produced in response to the virus. However, these antibody tests are not specific, antibodies can be produced by the body in response to a range of particles not just one virus, finding antibodies in an individual is supposed to demonstrate that the virus was present but these antibodies may have been produced in response to other things. Therefore the presence of, for example, measles antibody does NOT tell you that measles virus is necessarily present, which is how these tests can produce false positives. In addition even if these tests were accurate, antibodies to viruses do not inform whether the virus is the cause of the disease, just that the viral particle was present.

6.7.2 Viral DNA/RNA testing

Testing for viral DNA has not been carried out by isolating the virus first, (which remember we do have techniques for doing) instead pieces of DNA found in the diseased cells or fluids are multiplied up, using biochemical techniques called polymerase chain reactions. This DNA could in fact be from anywhere in the body and is never verified by comparing to real viral DNA because the real viruses in diseases have never been isolated. With no standard viral isolation we have no way of verifying whether theses multiplied pieces of DNA are from viruses or not.

6.7.3 Viral properties

Other biochemical properties of the virus are again assumed by taking the disease fluid and adding that to cells, which may cause, for example, cells to stick to each other (e.g. haemagglutinin). This is assumed to be the way the virus sticks to a cell and enters cells causing the illness. But again even though we have all kinds of elaborate hypotheses as to how this viral sticking occurs, we have never isolated these cells undergoing attachment and infection, and never photographed them using modern electron microscopy techniques.

Other reactions caused by enzymes in these disease fluids are again inferred as viral, for example neuraminidase reactions are said to be from the virus, but again these enzymes are common products of immune cells, for example in the lysosomal parts of the body's own white blood cells that are used to break down unwanted cell debris, poisons, and microbes.

Some drugs that are used to counteract the action of viruses (anti-virals) are in fact just neuraminidase inhibitors, which supposedly; reduce cell breakdown, viral entry and therefore viral replication. However recent research shows how neuraminidase activity actually enhances our own cellular immune activity, therefore anti-retrovirals thought to be inhibiting the virus may just be simple immune suppressors inhibiting our own immune cells. Suppressing our immune reactions with drugs will usually give initial relief but in the long-term reduces the body's ability to deal with the problem.

> *"...the results of the current study clearly indicate a slowdown influence of neuraminidase on apoptosis in peripheral blood lymphocytes. The study shows that neuraminidase decreased the level of apoptosis in blood lymphocytes and **increased their vitality**."*

Journal of Physiology & Pharmacology, 2007 (58) Suppl 5, 253-262

That is to say if neuraminidase increases our immune cell activity then anti-neuraminidase drugs (so-called anti-virals) will slow down our immune cell activity.

A web site publicising these issues www.klein-klein-aktion.de has been set up by an organisation in Germany, pushing health authorities to acknowledge the lack of scientific confirmation of these viral disease theories, their experience has been quite illuminating:

> *"We have sent our questions to the Health Officials, Social Ministers of the German states, University clinics, local Doctors groups, Federal Doctor groups, the Robert-Koch-Institute, the Paul-Ehrlich-Institute, Research establishments and the Health Ministry in Bonn. In our desperation we have also turned to many Public Health politicians, to the State parliaments of Baden Wurttemberg and Bavaria, to the Federal parliament and to the Chancellor's office. We have requested the Press for help. We have requested Doctors for help. We still haven't received a single clear answer to our specific questions.*

> *...The authorities refer to the evidence of a time in which the virus couldn't be isolated, presented, characterised and photographed because the necessary technology wasn't developed. Viruses were diagnosed on the basis of symptoms. One can reasonably guess from this that the concept Contagion = poison = virus from the 18th & 19th centuries was transferred onto the components of cells which in the 20th century are referred to as a virus. The astonishing thing is that these descriptions apparently emerge in the secondary literature and are drawn upon as an explanation for poisoning and vaccine damage.*

> *...Although Professor Forschepiepe and Dr Buchwald first made this proposal to the Ministry for Health and Hygiene in Bonn in 1961. Since then the authorities have provided us with hundreds of so-called "Virus pictures". The Biologists and micro-biologists to whom we have presented these pictures, have adjudicated that in every case these viruses are not characterised and isolated. Certainly these pictures concern cellular tissue-thin-sections and cellular tissue-cross-sections."*

In summary, many kinds of laboratory tests can infer the presence of disease for example, there are tests that will show the presence of 'prostate specific antigen' (PSA) which can be indicative of prostate cancer, but other proteins could give a false positive and there may be other reasons for the presence of PSA, therefore once we have that test result it is then imperative that we go back to the patient and look at his prostate to confirm whether or not there is a tumor. This is of course exactly what happens in cancer diagnosis, however the problem with viral research is that we have the 'inference' i.e. lots of tests to show what viruses could do, but the verification has been omitted; nobody is going back to isolate and electron micrograph the virus. Initially this was because we simply didn't have the technology but now we do, is it avoided because we could be opening up a veritable can of worms … or a can of nothing?

CHAPTER SEVEN

7 How suppressing mild illnesses can create more serious disorders?

What are the consequences of suppressing symptoms with medication; the immediate impact on the body and the resulting susceptibility to illnesses in the future?

> *"Most diseases are the result of medication which has been prescribed to relieve and take away a beneficent and warning symptom on the part of Nature."*
>
> Elbert Hubbard (19/06/1856 – 7/05/ 1915)
> American writer, publisher, artist, and philosopher

We have so far established that our toxins are eliminated by the normal everyday functions of the body; defecation, urination, perspiration and respiration. If toxins build at a greater rate than we are capable of eliminating them, then we experience symptoms of illness whereby the body increases the physical elimination of toxins and associated microbes including bacteria, fungus and viruses by:

> ➢ Vomiting and diarrhoea.
> ➢ Respiratory mucus with coughing, sneezing and nasal discharge.
> ➢ Increased sweating and urination, with increased concentration and odour.

We are aware that this situation has not been directly 'caused' by the microbe and that therefore these illnesses being described as infectious illnesses are misleading as to the real causes of disease. The response to increased toxins with an increase in physical elimination, may also involve white blood cells in the mucus; these specialised immune cells are able to break down toxins and pathogenic microbes (germs associated with disease) that have accumulated as a result of the increased toxicity.

It is important to realise that these symptoms are <u>not</u> a kind of physiological malfunction but they are a precise coordinated response to a build up of toxicity and a subsequent imbalance of microbes. Most of the holistic therapies are able to perceive the bigger picture. By taking a step back and including all the functions and symptoms of the individual, they are able to understand the purpose of symptoms.

This approach places almost all other therapies together and distinctly apart from orthodox drug therapy; hence they are often grouped together under the banner of alternative, but they are in fact many and varied. However this view is beginning to change even among many orthodox scientists, conventional scientists are in fact looking at symptoms as a positive response to trauma, responses that have evolved over millennia, and as questioned in The New Scientists Oct 23, 1993:

> *"Should we treat the symptoms of disease, or are they an aid to recovery?"*

The article goes on to comment on research being carried out by other scientists, claiming that:

> *"The underlying message is uncontroversial enough: human beings and their illnesses are the products of a long evolutionary history. Yet modern medicine, for all its high-technology treatments and preventive strategies, has so far largely ignored this fact."*

Randolph M Nesse (Medical Doctor and Professor at University of Michigan Medical School) and George C Williams (Professor Emeritus University of New York, Member of US National Academy of Science) have written the book *'Evolution and Healing'*. In referring to the symptoms of the body as 'evolved adaptations' they and others have coined the term 'Darwinian Medicine'.

The book charts the many examples of how the human physiology responds to environmental trauma and how the symptoms have evolved for the benefit of the patient.

For example, the benefits of diarrhoea in the evacuation of intestinal pathogens, how the vomiting in morning sickness can protect the developing foetus from toxins and the physiological response to a sprained joint, they ask:

- Are the symptoms an incidental consequence of the trauma, or an adaptation to promote healing?
- How is the sensation of pain produced? …And what is its role in the healing process?
- Therefore **what harmful consequences may result from stopping the symptoms?**

They go on to state…"Only by answering these questions can we choose the correct treatment."

7.1 Cured or suppressed

Realising that the symptoms of illness perform a necessary function for our survival, we arrive at one of the most significant elements in our understanding of health, illness and the treatment of disease. Once we appreciate how increased levels of toxicity within the digestive system would lead to an elimination response e.g. vomiting and/or diarrhoea, we are able to distinguish 'the response', (the vomiting and diarrhoea), from 'the trauma', (the toxins).

In orthodox medicine often the response itself is seen as the problem and the real causes are frequently ignored; we visit our doctor with the problem of vomiting and diarrhoea. From this perspective we would be tempted to try and stop the reaction, believing that the vomiting and diarrhoea are themselves the problems to be stopped. Many pharmaceutical drugs are designed to do just that and the sales of such drugs to the public and to health authorities, hinge on that basic premise. Selling more drugs relies on the ability to maintain the perspective that the symptom is a mal-function; whilst we are convinced the symptom is the problem (rather than indicative of a problem) then the solution lies in drug intervention capable of stopping the perceived problem.

So with the build up of toxins in the digestive tract leading to vomiting and diarrhoea we may be given an anti-emetic to stop the vomiting and imodium to stop the diarrhoea. However, from our wider perspective, knowing that the 'symptom' is a 'response' to the problem of intestinal toxicity, taking something to stop the reaction is **'suppressive'** of the person's attempt to correct the imbalance. The symptoms may have been stopped but the problem is not resolved and one of the central themes of a holistic approach to health care is the understanding of this concept of **suppression.**

We could, however, justify the uses of suppressive medication if we were concerned about the effects of our responses; the response itself could be extremely uncomfortable, the response could persist for too long and it may also lead to secondary complications. For example excessive vomiting and diarrhoea could lead to dehydration with subsequent loss of other functions, in addition to headaches, low blood pressure, electrolyte imbalance etc.

All of which are valid concerns, which would therefore lead us to addressing these issues, treatment from your health practitioner would be successful according to their understanding of the illness. We would have to address the problem of the build up of toxicity, perhaps stimulate the elimination response and at the same time support the general function by re-hydrating, replacing minerals etc. However, without a perspective of the purpose of the response and knowledge of the possibility of suppression, doctors are likely to suppress all responses without distinguishing which of them is a necessary part of the curative response. Suppressing vitally important reactions could of course lead to more severe consequences.

In fact the pharmaceutical intervention of physiological responses in that manner is really only justified in 'end-state' pathology, when in fact the patient is unable to react, or when the reactions have become detrimental to the patient, the medical profession does in fact excel in accident and emergency situations. However it is an unfortunate fact of orthodox medical intervention that they have taken the rationale for treating emergency situations, to treat virtually all other conditions.

With our example of toxicity within the digestive tract leading to vomiting and diarrhoea, suppression of the actual response would in fact increase the chances of an '**unsuccessful**' elimination and could therefore result in the very situation we are trying to avoid, recurrent symptoms and/or prolonged symptoms.

> **Pharmaceutical suppression increases the chances of the ultimate symptom scenario many doctors say they are trying to avoid.**

7.2 Consequences of Suppression

From our example of toxic build-up within the digestive tract and subsequent response of vomiting and diarrhoea, we may ask, what happens to our problem after effective suppression of our response? What happens to those toxins that we have been trying to eliminate with the vomiting and diarrhoea if we suppress the vomiting and diarrhoea? Quite clearly, these toxins can remain; attracting germs (microbes) and changing the nature of the germs that are normally present. With these microbes and toxins remaining within the digestive tract, they could poison the tissues and cells in that region of the body. Toxins may even build up and pass across the membrane of the digestive tract into the blood system where they would then have access to other internal organs.

The suppression of the body's attempt to 'eliminate', could therefore lead to more serious and/or more internal problems. To avoid this, the body's immune system will once again react, leading to either a recurrence of the vomiting and diarrhoea or will engage other systems in an attempt to detoxify, eliminate or limit the damage caused by these potential poisons.

7.3 The futility of the vaccine aspiration

Germs can only be associated with disease if other disease factors are present; toxins, dead or injured tissue, nutritional deficiencies including dehydration, compromised elimination and immune function often caused by pharmaceutical drug suppression.

If we are to eliminate certain microbes, but in the future suffer any deterioration in health, due to toxicity, injured or dead tissue, we would of course suffer from the symptoms of disease.

Because of the many varieties of germs and the ubiquitous nature of germs present in every aspect of our body and environment, any number of them could multiply in these disease conditions, some may contribute to the toxicity others are even helpful in the breakdown of unwanted material.

But disease cannot be simply eliminated even if we could effectively eliminate some microbes, the key to maintaining health would be in addressing the reasons as to why we become susceptible to the infectious disease state in the first place regardless of the germs in our environment.

With the failure of the body to address disease conditions and the added stress of pharmaceutical drug suppression, germs that are normally harmless in most people (Hib and meningococcal bacteria, polio, echo and coxsackie viruses) can invade the body's internal systems and multiply at the sites of toxicity, damage and inflammation.

The key to avoiding serious disorders such as paralytic poliomyelitis, meningitis, and encephalitis is in understanding how the body deteriorates to the point where some of the trillions of germs normally kept safely outside of the body are allowed into the internal organs and nervous system. The solution lies in the understanding of the function of symptoms in disease, the dangers of drug suppression and the role of germs in health & disease.

A more detailed look at this issue can be found in the follow-up book *'SomaWisdom - The Science of Health & Healing'* by Trevor Gunn

CHAPTER EIGHT

8 What are the real risks of vaccination?

The strategies of the priesthood in defending the human from attacking entities, create castles, weapons and creeds of conduct to protect us, but of course restrict and eventually kill us, imposing its belief system on the enemy it becomes the enemy, it even affects those that resist, for resistance is part of the problem.

The vaccine elements are injected into the body, past the body's normal lines of defence, (exceptions being the oral vaccines, polio being the most common, although the UK schedule has recently changed to an injectable form). There are many ways of injecting; intravenously, subcutaneously, intramuscularly etc, vaccines are not injected intravenously and so some medical professionals believe that vaccines are therefore not injected into the blood. However, all injections including the intramuscular and subcutaneous will give their contents direct assess to the blood system, as the skin, in all instances of injection, will be pierced and therefore the immune functions of the skin are by passed.

8.1 Vaccines bypass most of the immune system

Vaccine producers claim to be stimulating the immune system when clearly they are not; most of the immune system is by-passed. Vaccine producers are pre-occupied with stimulating blood antibody responses to viruses, microbes and toxins, which is in fact highly illogical given the following:

> We **do <u>not</u> know** how or whether a virus causes an illness, viral causation is still a theory, and yet we do know that poisoning a cell creates viruses, therefore vaccine promoters cannot say that they have found the cause of a disease when they find indirect evidence of genetic material thought to be from a virus.

> We **do <u>not</u> know** the best immune response to these pathogens, therefore why are vaccine producers so concerned with creating blood anti-bodies, when other systems may be far more important?

> We **<u>do</u> know** that in individuals with poor immune function; - AIDS, allergies, asthma and autoimmune disease - their immune response favours anti-body production instead of the cellular response. Therefore why are we trying to create anti-bodies and effectively mimic the situation of immune dysfunction?

> We **<u>do</u> know** that children incapable of producing antibodies overcome illnesses and obtain immunity far better than children with poor cellular immunity, if antibodies do not appear to be as important as the cellular response, why are we not concerned with stimulating cellular immunity but instead pre-occupied with creating anti-bodies?

The practice of vaccination for the purpose of creating blood anti-bodies is in fact highly questionable. However, if in fact vaccine promoters acknowledge that whatever the mechanism is for immunity, the hope is that the vaccine will stimulate a similar enough response to allow immune learning and a reduced susceptibility to future illness. Then the second point to consider is how similar to an illness is the response to vaccination?

Having injected the vaccine components into the blood, the stimulation of a blood immune response (generally considered to be the creation of antibodies) is often thought of as being sufficient to create immunity. However, regardless of what immune elements are stimulated in the blood, a **successful** immune response does **not** just require the formation of antibodies or any other immune cells within the blood system; a successful immune response necessarily involves the successful **elimination** of the toxins and microbes. Any health professional that thinks the mere production of antibodies is indicative of an effective immune response does not understand immune 'processes'.

> *Mario Clerci of the National Cancer Institute in the US suggests: ...that by looking at HIV positive patients i.e. the ones that are producing antibodies, we're looking at the immune failures.*

In fact most individuals that are vaccinated do not seem to respond at all with visible symptoms, for some this may be indicative of sufficient health and minimal sensitivity to the components of the vaccines, for others this could be indicative of an inability to eliminate toxins and therefore an increased immune load and greater susceptibility to future illness.

Essentially it is hoped that the vaccine will cause the body to create antibodies, even though, immunologists have to admit to not knowing the precise mechanism of the immune response to viruses, or for that matter any other pathogen.

The hope is of course that whatever the mechanism is, the action of the vaccine will stimulate a similar enough response in order to prime the body for any subsequent attack. But here we immediately run into significant problems, the injection of many vaccine pathogens alone actually stimulates little or no apparent immune response in the blood – antibodies or otherwise.

8.2 A spoon full of poison – helps the medicine go down

In fact, in order for some vaccines to stimulate the immune system to any significant degree a substance called an **adjuvant** is added to the vaccine contents. An Adjuvant is a chemical that will stimulate an immune response; it is therefore toxic to the human body and is effectively a **poison**. Without this poison the vaccine doesn't have a significantly measurable antibody response. The most common adjuvant is aluminium, a heavy metal with known toxic effects on the nervous system.

Why does the body <u>not</u> mount a significant immune response to the elements of the vaccine?

It does sound rather strange, that if we have made for example a diphtheria, tetanus, Hib meningitis, hepatitis B, DPT, Pediacel 5 in 1 vaccine, why does the body not produce a significant immune response to the elements of the vaccine without having to add another poison?

> Here we may come to the understanding that actually the live, attenuated or killed pathogen does not pose a significant or <u>apparent</u> threat to the human body; by the reactions, or rather lack of reaction, of the human body to these vaccine pathogens, it would appear that they may not be the real cause of illnesses.

> The lack of reaction to the vaccine pathogens may be as a result of changing the pathogen in the process of making the vaccine; it is possible that the vaccine components do not significantly mirror the real virus, microbe or toxin.

> In addition, illnesses in their natural form would arise from a natural build up of toxins and microbes on the outer membranes of your body or from an obvious injury. You would be alerted to a problem and would already be mounting an inflammatory response; infiltration of these elements into the blood will be quickly followed by a blood immune response that will make every attempt to eliminate these toxic elements. However a vaccine bypasses most of this response.

8.3 Trouble in the house – Poisons in the blood

An adjuvant, therefore, is a substance that helps and enhances the pharmacological effect of a drug or increases the ability of an antigen to stimulate the immune system. It is given because the vaccine contents alone do not stimulate a significant response on their own. In defence of the adjuvant, the pharmaceutical industries say that it is added so that they need less of the vaccine antigen, (the bacteria, virus or toxin in its changed form).

However, considering the toxicity of the adjuvant, why would you rather add adjuvant and not a little more vaccine antigen, given that the antigen i.e. the changed bacteria, virus or toxin is supposed to be rendered safe? Is it that these vaccine contents (antigens) are simply not recognised as an apparent threat to the body and therefore the question is; does the immune response to the vaccine really mimic the real disease situation sufficiently well enough to confer the much desired life-long immunity to the actual illness?

8.3.1 Aluminium

The adjuvant would be an obvious cause for concern, yet seems to go un-noticed as far as the possibility of creating adverse events from the vaccine. The most common adjuvant is aluminium, which is a known neurotoxin; there are dozens of studies that have implicated aluminium in the development of nervous system and brain disorders such as Alzheimer's disease.

> ➤ The mechanisms involved in the pathogenesis of the neurotoxicity associated with aluminium are numerous. (CNS Drugs. 2001; 15(9):691-9).

> ➤ Dr. Hugh Fundenburg, a biologist with nearly 850 papers in peer review journals, presented data at the 1997 International Vaccine Conference which shows that a person who takes 5 or more annual flu vaccine shots has increased the likelihood of

developing Alzheimer's disease by a factor of 10 over the person who has had 2 or fewer flu shots. When asked why, Dr. Fundenburg stated it is due to the mercury and aluminium build-up that are in many flu shots and in many other childhood vaccines. The gradual mercury and aluminium build-up in the brain causes eventual cognitive dysfunction.

➤ We know that traces of aluminium in the feed of preterm infants is associated with impaired neurological development, (N England J Med. 1997 Oct 9;337(15):1090-1) and yet children can often receive up to 3.75 mg of aluminium from vaccines during the first six months of life. (Pharmacol Toxicol 1992 Apr;70(4):278-80)

➤ Indeed even at the injection site of aluminium containing vaccines, reports since 1996 show that the pathological changes (disease changes of the skin and flesh) are greater than previously recognised (J Clinical Pathology (1996 Oct) 49(10):844-7).

➤ As reported earlier Dr Weil on the expert panel reviewing a study of the relationship of polyvalent vaccines and the increase in neurological disease, stated:

> "In relationship to aluminium, (an additive in many vaccines), being a nephrologist for a long time, the potential for aluminium and central nervous system toxicity was established by dialysis data. To think there isn't some possible problem here is unreal."

➤ Speaking of her autistic patients, Dr Stephanie Cave one time research specialist now a medical doctor in Louisiana:

> "You would be amazed at the devastation in their chemistries when you get down to the cellular level." She also said, "I think in later years we are going to

look back at aluminium the way we are looking at mercury now."

So what are the agreed safe levels of aluminium?

Until recently there were no upper safety levels set for environmental exposure, but the European Food Safety Association has newly recommended an upper level in dietary intake of 1mg per kg of body weight per week (22 May 2008). Acknowledging that 99.9% to 99.7% will be excreted through the gut and never enter the blood and internal systems of the body, but this absorption level can increase by as much as ten fold if other factors are present in the diet that aid assimilation.

Therefore the recommendation allows that a possible 3% of the upper safety limit could be absorbed into the body. A 6 month old child, maximum body weight 10 kg, would therefore have an upper safety limit of 3% of 10 mg aluminium per week having access to the internal body which is a **weekly maximum** of **0.3mg** yet a single injection can contain 2.5 times that at **0.85mg**, with a child receiving that in one day.

Are these levels in vaccines safe? It seems that the upper limits recommended for vaccines have been guessed and assigned by**... we don't know who...** as revealed by the transcripts from the National Vaccine Program Office Workshop on Aluminium in Vaccines, May 2000.

Dr. Gerber, National Institute of Health in fact asks the question:

> *"... the standard of 0.85 milligrams of aluminium per dose set forth in the Code of Federal Regulations, can you tell us where that came from and how that was determined?* "

Dr. Baylor appears qualified to answer that question, he is: Acting Deputy Director of the Office Of Vaccine Research and Review, and Associate Director for Regulatory Policy at the Centre for Biological Evaluation of Research at FDA... however his answer is somewhat revealing:

"Unfortunately, I could not. I mean, we have been trying to figure that out. We have been trying to figure that out as far as going back in the historical records and determining how they came up with that and going back to the preamble to the regulation. We just have been unsuccessful with that but we are still trying to figure that out."

So we are injecting neurotoxins into our children and adults, and the vaccine community does not know what levels are safe, but do in fact appear to be guessing at doses...this of course isn't science. As Dr. Martin Myers, Director of the National Vaccine Program Office, Department of Health and Human Services recognises and states in the same meeting:

"Perhaps the most important thing that I took away from the last meeting was that those of us who deal with vaccines have really very little applicable background with metals and toxicological research."

Scientists get scared

Neuroscientist Chris Shaw and a four scientist team from the University of British Columbia and Louisiana State University, conducted studies to test the possible impact of vaccines in the emergence of Gulf War Syndrome. Because Gulf War Syndrome looks a lot like; Parkinson's, amyotrophic lateral sclerosis and Alzheimer's, the neuroscientists had a chance to isolate a possible cause. All deployed troops were vaccinated with an aluminium hydroxide compound. Vaccinated troops who were not deployed to the Gulf developed similar symptoms at a similar rate, i.e. **illness developed whether they went to the Gulf or not**, therefore causation had to be due to a procedure they were all subjected to in their home country and not an issue in the Gulf itself.

The following comments were obtained by Pieta Woolley of Georgia Straight, Canada and published on 23-Mar-2006.

Shaw is most surprised that the research for his paper hadn't been done before. After 20 weeks studying vaccinated mice, the team found statistically significant increases in anxiety (38 percent); memory deficits (41 times the errors as in the sample group); and an allergic skin reaction (20 percent). Tissue samples after the mice were "sacrificed" showed neurological cells were dying. Inside the mice's brains, in a part that controls movement, 35 percent of the cells were destroying themselves.

"For 80 years, doctors have injected patients with aluminium hydroxide, an adjuvant that stimulates immune response. This is suspicious, either this [link] is known by industry and it was never made public, or industry was never made to do these studies by Health Canada. **I'm not sure which is scarier."**

"No one in my lab wants to get vaccinated," he said. **"This totally creeped us out. We weren't out there to poke holes in vaccines. But all of a sudden, oh my God-we've got neuron death!"** Shaw warns that "whether the risk of protection from a dreaded disease outweighs the risk of toxicity is a question that demands our urgent attention...I don't think the safety of vaccines is demarcated. How does a parent make a decision based on what's available? You can't make an intelligent decision...Conservatively, if one percent of vaccinated humans develop ALS from vaccine adjuvants, it would still constitute a health emergency."

It's possible that there are 10,000 studies that show aluminium hydroxide is safe for injections. But he **hasn't been able to find any that look beyond the first few weeks** of injection. If anyone has a study that shows something different, he said, please "put it on the table. That's how you do science."

Neuroscience research is difficult, Shaw said, because symptoms can take years to manifest, so it's hard to prove what caused the symptoms.

"To me, that calls for better testing, not blind faith."

This is certainly not the image of our knowledgeable vaccine promoters publicized by drug companies and health authorities; there is, of course, a huge divide between science, vaccine research and the public portrayal of vaccines.

8.3.2 Mercury

Alice in Wonderland...

Alice sighed wearily. 'I think you might do something better with the time,' she said, 'than waste it in asking riddles that have no answers.'

'If you knew Time as well as I do,' said the Hatter, 'you wouldn't talk about wasting it. It's him.'

'I don't know what you mean,' said Alice.

'Of course you don't!' the Hatter said, tossing his head contemptuously. 'I dare say you never even spoke to Time!'

'Perhaps not,' Alice cautiously replied: 'but I know I have to beat time when I learn music.'

'Ah! That accounts for it,' said the Hatter. 'He won't stand beating. Now, if you only kept on good terms with him, he'd do almost anything you liked with the clock. For instance, suppose it were nine o'clock in the morning, just time to begin lessons: you'd only have to whisper a hint to Time, and round goes the clock in a twinkling! Half-past one, time for dinner!'

('I only wish it was,' the March Hare said to itself in a whisper.) 'That would be grand, certainly,' said Alice thoughtfully: 'but then - I shouldn't be hungry for it, you know.'

'Not at first, perhaps,' said the Hatter: 'but you could keep it to half-past one as long as you liked.'

The expression mad as a hatter and the character in Lewis Carroll's *Alice in Wonderland* reflect a widely known phenomena of the 19th century. The term comes from an occupational disease in the manufacturers of top hats who used mercury compounds in the stiffening products for the felt. It has been known for many years that mercury is a cumulative poison causing, kidney and brain damage, with symptoms of trembling (known at the time as *hatter's shakes*), tooth loss and tooth decay, loss of co-ordination, difficult speech, anger, irritability, memory loss, depression, anxiety, paranoia and other personality changes. This was called *mad hatter syndrome* and is basically the symptoms of mercury poisoning.

We then, of course, have the much more publicised issue of the mercury content of vaccines. The mercury is in an antibiotic compound called Thiomersal added to vaccines to stop unwanted bacteria growing in the vaccine medium, it is used in the preparation and storage of some vaccines, (DPT, Tetanus, Hep.B, Flu, and Men.C, A vaccines).

It has been implicated as one of the major contributory factors in the many problems caused by vaccines, and in some countries it has now been reduced from some childhood vaccines, (though not completely removed as is often stated, it remains in concentrations that are still toxicological). And there has been no attempt at reduction in the Flu, Men A, C and Tetanus vaccines, where the thiomersal still remains in much greater concentrations.

Similarly the use of thiomersal continues unabated in most developing countries by the World Health Organisation, due to the higher cost of producing the less harmful mercury-reduced vaccines. Like aluminium, mercury is also a neurotoxin: When chemists subject nerve cells in Petri dishes to minute amounts of thiomersal, these cells die.

Drug testing - ignorance or deceit?

The mercury compound Thiomersal is used to stop the growth of unwanted bacteria in vaccines and was developed by the pharmaceutical company Eli Lilly in the 1920s. Until the 1990's many orthodox doctors and scientists trusted their assertion that thiomersal was safe, their declaration was however based on intentionally misleading experiments:

Dr. Mark A. Sircus Ac., OMD International Medical Veritas Association:

> …"Documents from the archives of Eli Lilly and Co., the original manufacturer of thimerosal, clearly demonstrates that the mercury-based vaccine preservative, implicated in a number of recent lawsuits as causing neurological injury to infants, was known as early as April 1930 to be dangerous.

> In its apparent eagerness to promote and market the product, in September 1930, **Eli Lilly secretly sponsored a "human toxicity" study on patients already known to be dying of meningococcal meningitis.** Andrew Waters of the Dallas-based law firm of Waters & Kraus stated that, "Lilly then cited this study repeatedly for decades as proof that thimerosal was of low toxicity and harmless to humans. They never revealed to the scientific community or the public the highly questionable nature of the original research.

> The tests were conducted in 1929 by a young researcher named K.C. Smithburn who injected 22 human subjects (who were already dying) with a 1 percent solution and then pronounced that all the patients were reported "**without ill effect.**" That they all died was never mentioned. "It's apparent that Eli Lilly didn't want to do the study themselves because it's apparent that there were enormous ethical problems with injecting people -- even people dying of meningitis -- with mercury," Waters said. "What Smithburn did was wrong, because he agreed to do the study for Eli Lilly, and not only did he agree to do it, but he agreed to give them results that he knew were flawed."

> There simply are no words that can be used to describe what Eli Lilly & Co., and then other pharmaceutical companies perpetuated through decades of use of a highly toxic compound like thimerosal. And there is no ethical explanation for current and former American administrations that have either tried or succeeded in providing protection to Lilly and other pharmaceutical companies from lawsuits for damages done to children from the use of their products."

The safety of thiomersal was based on an experiment using dying patients with damaged and inflamed nervous systems; the experiment found that no harmful effect, nor indeed any change, could be noted when injecting thiomersal in these meningitis patients, because …they already had severely damaged immune and nervous systems and… were dying anyway.

It was like taking a bale of straw already ablaze with flames and throwing on a lighted match, the lighted match did nothing… it was of course burning anyway.

The effects of mercury as a neurotoxin have in fact been known for many years. <u>Kamila K Padlewska, MD</u>, Assistant Professor, Department of Dermatology and Venereology, Warsaw Medical School, Poland has this to say about 'Acrodynia', a syndrome common until the 1960's:

> Now a rare disease, 'acrodynia' primarily affects young children. The symptoms of irritability, photophobia, pink discoloration of the hands and feet, and polyneuritis (inflammation of the nerves) can be attributed to chronic exposure to mercury.

> The most frequent sources of mercury prior to the legislated removal of the heavy metal from these preparations were calomel-containing anthelminthics, laxatives, diaper rinses, teething powders, fungicides in paint, repeated gamma-globulin injections, termite-protected wood (mercury bichloride), watch batteries (ie, via ingestion), mercurial antibacterial ointments, mercurial skin-lightening creams, and dental amalgam. The legislated removal of this heavy metal corresponded to the virtual disappearance of acrodynia...

Because the metal can be stored in the body to some extent and intolerance may develop long after exposure, morbid symptoms may appear weeks or months after the exposure or drug administration, with its cause escaping recognition.

According to Dr. Boyd E. Haley, Chairman of Chemistry Department, Kentucky University:

> "Any competent biochemist would look at the structure of thiomersal and identify it as a potent enzyme inhibitor. What is surprising is that the appropriate animal and laboratory testing was not done on the vaccines containing thiomersal (and aluminum) before the government embarked on a mandated

vaccine program that exposed infants to the levels of thiomersal that occurred."

Part of the existing problem we are told therefore resides in the lack of clinical studies carried out on thiomersal; however we have to acknowledge that much of the trouble also rests in the inability to acknowledge existing safety data for mercury toxicity. There has been upper safety limits set to limit excessive mercury exposure to individuals; it is banned from antibiotic preparations, fungicides, paints, cosmetics, and more recently dental amalgam in some countries, yet large doses are allowed in many of our vaccines.

8.3.3 Massive over-dosing

The USA Environmental Protection Agency has set an upper safety limit of mercury exposure to 0.1 mcg per kg body weight per day. A child of 6 months old with a maximum weight of 10 kg should therefore **not** be exposed to more than **1 mcg of mercury/day.**

Yet a single DPT vaccine contains a whopping **25 mcg of mercury** at least 25 times the level already set by the EPA in just one single injection. Most children are in fact given **3 shots** before the age of 6 months old.

Even more problematic was the fact that, vaccine promoters and other scientists failed to calculate the mercury load that would be injected into children by adding up the total mercury content of all the subsequent vaccines and additional boosters given to children within the space of a few months. These problems are further exacerbated when we learn that mercury is eliminated from the body by its attachment to bile from the liver, however children can only produce bile from the age of 6 months and would have great difficulty eliminating mercury before that age.

In 1999, Dr Neal Halsey, who heads the Hopkins Institute for Vaccine Safety said:

"My first reaction was simply disbelief, which was the reaction of almost everybody involved in vaccines…

"In most vaccine containers, thiomersal is listed as a mercury derivative, a hundredth of a percent. And what I believed, and what everybody else believed, was that it was truly a trace, a biologically insignificant amount. My honest belief is that if the labels had had the mercury content in micrograms, this would have been uncovered years ago. But the fact is, no one did the calculation"

The closer we look into this issue the more problematic it becomes, Dr Tim O'Shea in his book 'The Sanctity of Human Blood' explains:

"In the U.S., EPA mercury toxicity studies have involved contamination from fish, air, and other environmental sources. The mercury in vaccines, however, is in the form of thiomersal, which is 50 times more toxic than plain old mercury…

Reasons for this include:

➢ *Injected mercury is far more toxic than ingested mercury.*
➢ *There's no blood-brain barrier in infants.*
➢ *Mercury accumulates in brain cells and nerves.*
➢ *Infants don't produce bile, which is necessary to excrete mercury.*

"Thiomersal becomes organic mercury: Once it is in nerve tissue, it is converted irreversibly to its inorganic form. Thiomersal is a much more toxic form of mercury than one would get from eating open-sea fish; it has to do with the difficulty of clearing thiomersal from the blood.
Without a complete blood-brain barrier, an infant's brain and spinal cord are sitting ducks. Once in the nerve cells, mercury

is changed back to the inorganic form and becomes tightly bound. Mercury can then remain for years, like a time-release capsule, causing permanent degeneration and death of brain cells."

8.3.4 Introducing autism

In the USA, April 2000, at the congressional hearing on autism and vaccines, the Sallie Bernard study of vaccines and mercury toxicity has been cited as one of the main reasons Congress began to see the obvious correlation between the rise of autism and the introduction of thiomersal in vaccines.

> ➤ Autism was first described in 1943 among children born in the 1930s; Thiomersal was first introduced into vaccines in the 1930s. The subsequent increase in autistic rates parallels the introduction of new vaccines containing thiomersal.

> ➤ The age at which autistic symptoms are first noticed in children and the ages of the subsequent increase in their autistic symptoms closely correlates to the times at which thiomersal containing vaccines are introduced throughout their lives in the typical vaccination schedule.

> ➤ Every major symptom of autism matches the symptoms of documented cases of mercury poisoning: Social deficits, shyness, depression, anxiety, impaired face recognition, irrational fears, aggression, lack of eye contact, attention problems, loss of speech, sound sensitivity or loss of hearing, light sensitive, blurred vision, jerking rocking circling motions, lack of coordination, lack of understanding, self injurious behaviour, staring, unprovoked crying, sleep difficulties, incontinence, digestive disturbances, anorexia.

> ➤ The biological and biochemical characteristics of the nervous system and immune system affected by mercury poisoning are

the same as in autism, in addition both autistic patients and victims of mercury poisoning show low glutathione and sulphate levels, purine and pyrimidine metabolic disruption as well as mitochondrial dysfunction.

➤ When mercury elimination techniques are used to remove mercury not only from the extracellular fluid but from within the cells, symptoms of autism show a marked improvement.

➤ There is an inherited predisposition to the effects of mercury poisoning just as with autism, with a higher than expected incidence in other siblings. Therefore not all individuals are affected in the same manner.

➤ Studies of mercury poisoning in animals and humans consistently report greater effects in males than in females, autism seems to affect more males than females.

These phenomena have been studied by David Ayoub MD who is a board-certified radiologist and associate professor at Southern Illinois University School of Medicine in Springflield Illinois he similarly asserts that every major characteristic of mercury poisoning in a child matches the syndrome of autism.

The rate of autism has increased in the 1930's from being a new and rare phenomenon to 1 in 2000 before the 1970's, which equates to **50 in 100,000**, note that a **polio epidemic is 35 in 100,000**, and according to research conducted by G Baird et al published in the Lancet 2006; (368: 210–15), studies reveal that as many as 1 in 86 children are on the autistic spectrum, that equates to approximately **1,160 per 100,000.** 'Autistic spectrum disorders' being the newer term recognised by the WHO, describes the disease syndrome as characterized by widespread abnormalities of social interactions and communication, as well as severely restricted interests and highly repetitive behavior.

8.3.5 Further evidence incriminating vaccines in autism

The official line is that vaccines are not implicated in autism with many officials choosing not to address the evidence by simply saying there is no evidence; however the walls are beginning to close in, on those in denial. One simple study would be to compare autism rates in the vaccinated and unvaccinated.

Generation Rescue commissioned an independent opinion research firm, Survey USA of Verona NJ, to conduct a survey in nine counties within California and Oregon. Generation Rescue chose to closely mirror the methodology the CDC uses to establish national prevalence for neurological disorders such as ADHD and autism, also matching the age range used by CDC. When asked are the parent responses used in the survey a reliable indicator of a child's diagnostic status? According to Dr. Laura Schieve, co-author of the CDC's national phone survey study, in discussing the CDC's two phone surveys on autism prevalence, "the consistency of prevalence estimates across the two surveys supports high reliability or reproducibility of parental report of autism and reliability is one important component of validity."

And what were the results of that study?

> "We surveyed over 9,000 boys in California and Oregon and found that ___vaccinated___ *boys had a* ___155%___ *greater chance of having a neurological disorder* like ADHD or autism than unvaccinated boys." -Generation Rescue, June 26, 2007
> *"Generation Rescue is a small non-profit organization. For less than $200,000, we were able to complete a study that the CDC, with an $8 billion a year budget, has been unable or unwilling to do. We think the results of our survey lend credibility to the urgent need to do a larger scale study to compare vaccinated and unvaccinated children for neurodevelopmental outcomes."*

In addition there are now details of a settlement reached in 2007, disclosed in March 2008, as the first autism case where United States government lawyers agreed that it was triggered by childhood vaccinations. Hannah Poling v. U.S. Department of Health and Human

Services. This concession was granted without any courtroom proceedings, effectively preventing any public hearing discussing what happened to Hannah and why. Details were revealed in The New York Times, March 8, 2008.

> "Hannah, of Athens, Georgia USA, was 19 months old and developing normally in 2000 when she received five shots against nine infectious diseases. Two days later, she developed a fever, cried inconsolably and refused to walk. Over the next seven months she spiralled downward, and in 2001 she was given a diagnosis of autism."

United States government officials state that this is a very rare case of vaccine damage due to the nature of a 'rare' mitochondrial disorder that Hannah was suffering from, the implication is that most if not all other autistic cases do not satisfy these conditions. It was then referred to as a mitochondrial dysfunction, i.e. not as bad as a 'disorder' because in fact Hannah had **no symptoms before the vaccines**.

However in acknowledging the impact of vaccines in these individuals, evidence is emerging that suggests mitochondrial disorders among autistic children are not rare at all. At the American Academy of Neurology 60th Annual Meeting (April 2008), a retrospective analysis of 41 children with autistic spectrum disorders who were being evaluated for suspected mitochondrial disease showed that 32 (**78%**) had defects in skeletal muscle oxidative phosphorylation (OXPHOS) enzyme function and 29 of 39 (**74%**) harbored abnormalities in the OXPHOS proteins, both indicative of mitochondrial dysfunction. Far from being rare this one study suggests that more children on the autistic spectrum have this disorder, than do not.

Stop Press: 20th Feb 2009 – 10 year old Bailey Banks awarded damages after ruling concluded MMR vaccine caused Encephalomyelitis and subsequent autism.
8.3.6 Then we add the two together; mercury and aluminium

According to Dr Donald W Miller physician and teacher of cardiac surgery at the University of Washington, School of Medicine:

> "Another important factor with regard to mercury on the mind, which officials at the CDC, FDA and the professors in the IOM do not consider, is synergistic toxicity - mercury's enhanced effect when other poisons are present. A small dose of mercury that kills 1 in 100 rats and a dose of aluminium that will kill 1 in 100 rats, when combined have a striking effect: **_all the rats die_**. Doses of mercury that have a 1 percent mortality will have a 100 percent mortality rate if some aluminium is there".

Dr. Boyd Haley at the University of Kentucky, conducting experiments to determine if aluminium would increase the toxicity of very low levels of thiomersal, reported:

> "The results were unequivocal: The presence of aluminium dramatically increased the rate of neuronal death caused by thiomersal. Therefore, the aluminium and thiomersal combination found in vaccines produces a toxic mixture that cannot be compared to situations where thiomersal alone was the toxic exposure."

Remember Dr Neal Halsey in 1999, who heads the Hopkins Institute for Vaccine Safety:

> "My honest belief is that if the labels had had the mercury content in micrograms, this would have been uncovered years ago. But the fact is, no one did the calculation"

The fact is, we have done the calculations, and as a result of the work of independent researchers and campaigners bringing this evidence to the attention of government officials, some vaccines previously containing high doses of thiomersal have had their mercury levels dramatically reduced, after 70 years of injecting mercury into children the authorities decided to do something about it. Yet these authorities have still not once acknowledged the role of vaccines in cases of neurological damage in vaccine victims.

However, once the decision had been made to reduce these levels of mercury, in some vaccines, it took an additional number of years to achieve because the pharmaceutical companies were allowed to use old stocks of vaccines containing the high levels of mercury. The reduced level still leaves mercury present in quantities of about 0.3 – 0.5 mcg of mercury, a quantity that is left over from the manufacturing process and this does not of course address the issue of Aluminium toxicity.

With more than three of these vaccines in a young child this still reaches over the upper safety limits of mercury in the form of thiomersal which still does not take into account the more dangerous issue of thiomersal mercury in a vaccine:

> It is injected past the bodies' natural lines of defence.
> It is organic in nature therefore gaining easier access to the internal tissues.
> Children before 6 months old cannot eliminate mercury efficiently as they are not yet able to produce bile.

In addition there are still vaccines in use that contain a huge 25mcg of mercury that are currently given to children and adults, mainly the tetanus and some flu vaccines, which the British government are considering adding to the childhood vaccine schedule. And the WHO still uses the old vaccines in developing countries, as the reduced mercury-containing single vial shots are considered to be too expensive.

The fact that most health authorities missed the opportunity to clinically assess the toxicity of vaccines or to inform their health professionals of the exact nature and content of vaccines, and in addition failed to notice the adverse effects of these vaccines in individuals - until independent researchers brought these facts to light, illustrates how the very authorities in whom we entrust our health are either completely incompetent or for whatever reason have more Important concerns than the health and wellbeing of their public.

8.4 Immune Complexes

Moving on to the issue of the antigen, i.e. the actual microbe or toxin that we are vaccinating with, (e.g. the measles virus in the measles vaccine or the tetanus toxin of the tetanus vaccine etc), one problem associated with injecting such elements into the body (as well as the problems associated with the vaccine poisons), is the fact that they do attract antibodies to them thereby forming immune complexes.

Most of us think that creating antibodies in the blood that attaches to the foreign antigens is actually what we want; indeed the measure of a successful vaccine has historically been evaluated by the mere production of antibodies themselves. Antibodies that are able to attach to the vaccine elements that we are injecting, however, immunologists know that this is not the complete story.

These antibodies that attach to foreign antigens in the blood do so for a reason; to attract other immune cells that are able to breakdown and eliminate those potential poisons and pathogens, (pathogens = disease causing agents). These antibody antigen complexes (conjoined lock and key combinations) if not eliminated from the body, can become lodged in the small capillaries of any organ; this mechanism is extremely significant in the formation of kidney disease, brain disorders and other vascular illnesses.

> "Immune complexes of this nature can also be formed in people by simple vaccination procedures...There are now ample reasons for believing that any antigen capable of eliciting the formation of a precipitating antibody, and hence a soluble immune complex can form the basis of serious immune injury. Bacteria, viruses, chemicals and drugs are certainly candidates

in this important group of diseases." (Advances in Clinical
Immunology – R.Schwartz)

It would therefore be imperative that such immune complexes are
eliminated from the body, this 'anti-body antigen' complex **is supposed
to be eliminated**; that is the purpose of the immune response to such
foreign elements in the blood... inactivation **and elimination**. However
vaccine policy has in fact <u>no focus</u> on this elimination aspect at all; the
entire edifice of vaccination rests on the naive assumption that the
mere production of antibodies is indicative of an effective and therefore
desirable immune response, which therefore brings us to the next
predicament.

8.5 The Butterfly Effect

From studying complex systems, of which the human body is one,
scientists realise that small deviations or errors in calculations, in one
place, at one time, can have devastating effects in other parts at a later
date... The idea was light-heartedly known as the 'Butterfly Effect' ... a
butterfly stirring in China could create a storm one month later in
America.

This is however a very real problem when trying to calculate the
outcome of interventions in complex systems, none more so than the
effects of viral particles and poisons contained in vaccines on the
multifarious and intricate workings of the human body. So far we have
looked at the more predictable outcomes of vaccines; however,
scientists are simply at a loss to predict the effect that these vaccine
components will have in the long term... the Butterfly Effect. With the
process of vaccination, the small changes in human biochemistry
caused by the injection of unknown viral elements past the body's
normal lines of immune defence is inevitably a huge pharmaceutical
experiment, the outcome of which will only be known by the results of
prolonged, comprehensive and conscientious research.

8.5.1 Vaccine contaminant viruses

As the mechanisms of cellular research have become more and more sophisticated we are now able to observe effects that were hitherto unpredictable and imperceptible, for example, in 1960 contaminant viral particles were found in the inactivated polio vaccine. These vaccine viruses were grown on 'Simian' monkey kidney cells; hence the contaminant virus was labeled 'Simian Virus 40' (SV-40). This virus was found at the site of cancers that had developed in individuals after they had been vaccinated with the polio vaccine and therefore the vaccine was implicated as the cause of certain cancers. After investigations, inevitable cover-ups and denial, it was eventually acknowledged and the vaccine production method was changed from the simian monkey to the African Green monkey kidney cells.

However despite this new production, there was still evidence of contaminant viruses in the new polio vaccine, Dr John Martin, virologist and one time FDA scientist writes of this new vaccine:

> *"Persisting concerns regarding contaminating viruses in the live polio vaccine (of African Green Monkeys) led in 1972 to a joint study between the vaccine manufacturer and the United States Food and Drug Administration (FDA)."*

The results of this study showed that contaminant viruses could still be found using more sophisticated techniques but not by the techniques used by most standard protocols prevalent at that time, however...

> *"No changes in testing methodology were imposed, nor was the scientific community alerted to the findings. An excuse that was subsequently offered was that all such information about the study was deemed to be proprietary."*

Effectively the results of such studies were deemed to be the concerns of **pharmaceutical companies <u>only</u>**, (*"...deemed to be proprietary"*), not even other scientists much less members of the vaccinated public were privy to such information.

Dr Martin conducting further research, found that in some patients with complex neurological diseases, viruses isolated from them would evoke no inflammatory responses, the body apparently made no attempt to eliminate them, they were then termed 'Stealth Viruses' because of their ability to operate within the body undetected by the immune system. These viruses have been found in people with chronic fatigue syndrome, attention deficiency disorder, autism and other brain and nervous system conditions.

What is the role of these stealth viruses in pathology? We are already aware of the difficulty in ascribing the cause of disease to any specific virus; we know that they are, in many instances, probably the result of our own cellular breakdown. Hence viruses are species specific, each animal, insect, plant and bacteria have their own specific viruses. The problem with these so-called stealth viruses however, is that they are human in origin but then they are subsequently replicated on animal tissue, from which they are then injected into our bodies in the form of vaccines, many viruses in vaccines are now no longer human viruses.

We now know that these viruses have the capacity to assimilate genes from the cells on which they are grown, thereby having a combination of human and animal genes; in addition they are able to incorporate genes from bacterial contaminants and so far the cellular genes identified within the stealth virus also include a gene with potential oncogenic (cancer causing) activity.

Dr Martin commenting on the issue of stealth viruses...

> ...Human and animal viruses with bacterial sequences represent a novel life form that has been christened 'viteria'. The recombination of viral, bacterial and cellular genes within broadly infectious viteria is clearly of major medical and Public Health significance.

In an article published in the July 1995 issue of Clinical and Diagnostic Virology, Martin and his colleagues describe how they conducted DNA and amino acid sequence comparisons on such contaminant stealth viruses:

> "...The findings implicate the African green monkey as the probable source of the virus isolated from this CFS patient."...
> "...The potential introduction of pathogenic viral variants into humans through the use of African green monkey-derived cell lines in live virus vaccine production should be evaluated."

Dr John Martin a legitimate and respected research scientist found evidence of contaminants in vaccines, contaminants that could cause many kinds of illnesses, of which cancer has been one; however he suddenly found that the authorities were actively turning a blind eye. After years of further research he discovered that an FDA Reform Bill, was being considered by Congress in 1997. Dr Martin suggested that the bill include the provision that:

> "If a safety issue is identified in the regulation of a biological product, then Industry will waive its proprietary protection so that the information could be made available to the scientific community." The suggestion was well received by the counsel for the House Commerce Committee. It was soon dropped, however, when support was not forthcoming from Industry, FDA or the American Medical Association (AMA).

Dr Martin thought he could enrol the help of an AMA lobbyist, speaking on behalf of doctors; maybe they could bring pressure to bear on the government to introduce legislation compelling the research of drug companies to be made available to other scientists and doctors, Dr Martin was disappointed however...

In speaking with an AMA lobbyist, I understood they "would not want the public to know that their doctors were not in the knowledge loop"

The AMA, i.e. the United States association of medical doctors, felt they were in no position to start pressurising the government for such change as they would not want the public to know that they did not have access to such information in the first place...

We do not want you the public to know... that even we don't know.

The American Medical Association

Dr Martin was to uncover further resistance to the issue of dealing with contaminant viruses in vaccines, from his own research he knew they were there. After years of working in other laboratories and some time working in the FDA he wanted to know if scientists producing the polio vaccine were still finding contaminant viruses. Answers to such questions, as we know, are hidden from scientists and doctors, after identifying himself as 'just' an interested parent he was able to find out that contaminants were in fact still being found and most surprisingly he began to expose a web of deceit covering the fact that FDA officials would actually rather <u>not</u> know.

"I once asked industry personnel involved in polio vaccine production whether they were still encountering SCMV (contaminant virus) in polio vaccine production lots. After some hesitation that disappeared as we all identified ourselves as parents, the straightforward answer was "not infrequently." Armed with this information I again requested of an FDA official to please use modern techniques such as the polymerase chain reaction (PCR) to screen polio vaccine lots for SCMV. "We would not know what to do with a positive result" was his answer.

8.5.2 Vaccines and autoimmune disease

The American Physician Dr Harold Buttram recognises a parallel with the stealth virus phenomena observed by Dr Martin and the work of Dr Vijendra Singh published in 'Clinical Immunology & Immunopathology' (Vol 88 (1); 1998: 105-108).

> *Although scientific evidence has not yet reached the standards of proof, one pioneer researcher in this area, Dr. Vijendra Singh with the University of Michigan, has published a report of a study in which he found that a large majority of autistic children tested had antibodies to brain tissue, in the form of antibodies to myelin basic protein. He also found a strong correlation between myelin basic protein antibodies and antibodies to measles, mumps, and rubella (almost all of the children had been immunized with MMR, and none had had these diseases before).*

> *This study confirms the results of a similar study published in The Lancet in 1998 by Dr. Andrew Wakefield of the Royal Free hospital in London, showing a link between MMR vaccination and Crohn's disease of the bowel and autism.*

> *If the MMR vaccine were causing an autoimmune reaction involving the brains of autistic children, what would be the mechanism? Although research in this area is in its infancy, as previously mentioned, we do know some things. Both the measles and mumps fractions of the MMR vaccine are cultured in chick embryo tissue. As purely genetic material, viruses are highly susceptible to the process of "jumping genes," in which they may incorporate genetic material from the tissues in which they are cultured. Once this genetic material of chick origin is introduced into the child, it may set in motion an immunologic battleground, a process that the work of Dr. Singh would tend to confirm.*

In summary, it is possible that either the MMR or the oral polio vaccines, by mechanisms described above may induce a process of encephalitis or brain inflammation, which may be highly prevalent but as yet rarely recognized for its true nature.

There have also been studies that acknowledge the role of vaccines in causing the autoimmune disease Lupus and so the phenomenon is a known consequence of vaccination.

8.5.3 Adjuvant Squalene and autoimmune disease

Squalene is a naturally occurring oil found in humans and other animals and is especially concentrated around the nerve cells of the body and the brain. The WHO on their website www.who.int confirms that squalene is being used as an adjuvant in vaccines:

> ➢ *Since 1997, an influenza vaccine (FLUAD, Chiron) which contains about 10 mg of squalene per dose, has been approved in health agencies in several European countries. Squalene is present in the form of an emulsion and is added to make the vaccine more immunogenic.*

> ➢ *Squalene is being added to improve the efficacy of several experimental vaccines including pandemic flu and malaria vaccines which are being developed*

World Health Organisation

But once squalene is injected, along with the other vaccine components, the body is alerted to squalene as a toxin, thereby creating anti-bodies and initiating immune reactions against it. These antibodies and immune responses can then 'cross-react' to our own naturally occurring squalene, thereby causing a cascade of inflammatory destruction of our own nervous systems. Once this reaction starts it may never stop, as the body continually replaces the natural component that the immune system is now trained to destroy and eliminate, as with the cases of autoimmune illnesses like multiple sclerosis and others.

Gary Matsumoto writing in his book 'Vaccine – A' explains the situation further:

> "As any immunologist will tell you, the way an antigen encounters the immune system makes all the difference. You can eat squalene - no problem as it is an oil the body can easily digest. But studies in animals and humans show that injecting squalene will galvanize the immune system into attacking it, which can produce a self-destructive cross reaction against the same molecule in the places where it occurs naturally in the body - and where it is critical to the health of the nervous system."

> ...The real problem with using squalene, of course, is not that it mimics a molecule found in the body; it is the same molecule..."So what American scientists conceived as a vaccine booster was another "nano-bomb", instigating chronic, unpredictable and debilitating disease. When the NIH (National Institutes of Health) argued that squalene would be safe because it is native to the body, just the opposite was true. Squalene's natural presence in the body made it one of the most dangerous molecules ever injected into man!

> ...scientists in the United States are now literally invested in squalene. Army scientists who developed the second generation anthrax vaccine have reputations to protect and licensing fees to reap for the army and worldwide rights to develop and commercialize the new recombinant vaccine for anthrax."

Unfortunately there is a very clear pattern emerging in researching vaccine side-effects, one in which the many legitimate research scientists discovering demonstrable risks associated with vaccines, find themselves sidelined and ostracised from governing health institutes, facing persistent denials as to the existence of any problems associated with vaccines. In such a climate it is difficult for members of the public, professional and otherwise, to reach informed conclusions about the safety and effectiveness of vaccines. However by piecing together the available evidence it is possible to do just that.

CHAPTER NINE

9 Are the authorities telling you everything they know about the dangers of vaccines?

We shall look at one more example of how health officials have been dealing with the question of the harmful effects of vaccines by looking at the issue of mercury in the vaccines that are routinely given to children. There is currently a debate raging as to the possible adverse effects of mercury in vaccines, more specifically on the neurological development (brain and nervous system) of young children.

Many physicians, scientists and those within the pharmaceutical industry know that vaccines can cause all kinds of serious adverse effects and can, although rarely, kill. There are, however, more subtle developmental syndromes increasing in the developed world, affecting many more individuals, these syndromes have also been linked to vaccination and many, suspect the mercury in some vaccines could be partly responsible.

In the USA the main medical institutions responsible for advising on public health policy, for reviewing and conducting research are: The Institute of Medicine (IOM), The Centre for Disease Control (CDC), The American Medical Association (AMA) and The American Academy of Paediatrics (AAP), Advisory Committee on Immunisation Practises (ACIP), National Immunization Program (NIP).

All are assuring people that the benefits of vaccines far outweigh the problems and more specifically that the mercury in vaccines is safe. Much of this recent display of confidence in the safety of mercury in vaccines relates to a two-phase study completed in 2003. This study consisted of the observation of health records, (Computerized Health Maintenance Organization Databases), which are recorded incidences of symptoms and illnesses reported by physicians to the health authorities.

From these records it may be possible to see if there are any correlations between the rise of certain illnesses known to be associated with mercury toxicity and the increase in the use of mercury containing vaccines. The results of their observations were published in Pediatrics, 112:1039-1048; the conclusions noted in the report stated that the study failed to find consistent associations between thiomersal containing vaccines and neurodevelopmental disorders.

The reported conclusions of this study have caused considerable controversy, with some outrage among the general public and those caring for friends and family with suspected vaccine damage. There is a growing frustration and distrust of the authorities as they appear to have covered up the initial findings of the study.

9.1 The Simpsonwood Meeting

A secret closed meeting on the subject of the original study was held in Simpsonwood, Georgia 7-8th June 2000. This was attended by members of the CDC and other health organizations from the USA and around the world, as well as representatives from the vaccine manufacturers. The transcript of this meeting has recently been obtained under the Freedom of Information Act, the content of which highlights many of the problems surrounding the assessment of vaccine safety and effectiveness.

Certainly recorded statements from the representatives of the various health agencies would give cause for concern. Dr Clements of the World Health Organisation (WHO):

> *"And I really want to risk offending everyone in the room by saying that perhaps this study should not have been done at*

all, because the outcome of it could have, to some extent, been predicted and we have all reached this point now where we are left hanging…"

9.2 Vaccines linked to brain & nervous system disorders

There was agreement that the study pointed to a legitimate correlation between some neurodevelopmental problems and the use of mercury containing vaccines, but nobody could conclude to any certainty whether it was the mercury or some other component of the vaccine as Dr Verstraeten the lead author of the study sates:

> *"Finally, and this may be the toughest one of all, how do we know that it is a Thimerosal effect? Since all vaccines* (in this study) *are Thimerosal containing, how do we know that it's not something else in the vaccines such as aluminum or the antigens?"*
>
> Dr Verstraeten

There was indeed a sense of shock in the findings, Dr Verstraeten and his team had carried out an enormous amount of detailed work, highly praised by all of the various delegates at the meeting. There could of course be all kinds of reasons for the apparent association between the use of vaccines and neurodevelopmental disorders. In fact there was always the possibility that the findings were somehow wrong, that there were inaccuracies due to reporting and diagnosis or just a chance correlation that could not be replicated. But of course as far as possible, all of these confounding factors were accounted for and the more stringent the criteria were applied the more significant became the results.

Given all of the possible confounding factors, what were Dr Verstraeten's thoughts as to the legitimacy of the findings of a link between mercury containing vaccines and neurodevelopmental disorders, what they refer to as their 'signal'; could the correlation between vaccine and neurological disorder go, if they took into account these other factors, (could the 'signal' go)?

> To me the bottom line is well; there are some things that just will never go away. If you make it go away here, it will pop up again there. So the bottom line is okay, our signal will simply not just go away.

Some experts at the meeting were not at all surprised at the findings and suggested that this is not just a simple issue of toxicity level, but an effect that will differ according to age of vaccination and consequently the developmental stage of the child when the toxic threshold is reached. Age may therefore have a two-fold effect, the younger child may be more neurologically sensitive and will also be less able to eliminate and neutralize the toxin.

Dr Weil on the expert panel:

> "...from all of the other studies of toxic substances, the earlier you work with the central nervous system, the more likely you are to run into a sensitive period for one of these effects, so that moving from one month or one day of birth to six months of birth changes enormously the potential for toxicity. There is just a host of neuro-developmental data that would suggest that we've got a serious problem."

Dr Weil also stated

> "In relationship to aluminium, (an additive in many vaccines), being a nephrologist for a long time, the potential for aluminium and central nervous system toxicity was established by dialysis data. To think there isn't some possible problem here is unreal."

According to the lead author of the study the question was then asked, let's suppose that there is a connection between mercury and neurodevelopmental disorders how plausible is it that mercury could cause these problems, from what we already know about mercury toxicity?

Dr. Brent:	*If it is true, which or what mechanisms would you explain the finding with?*
Dr. Verstraeten:	*You are asking for biological plausibility?*
Dr. Brent:	*Well, yes.*
Dr Verstraeten:	*When I saw this, and I went back through the literature, **I was actually stunned by what I saw**, because I thought it is plausible.*

We therefore have our lead researcher convinced that there is a legitimate link between neurodevelopmental disorders and the afore mentioned vaccines and that the biological mechanism is plausible, although nobody could be sure that this was due to the mercury and not some other component of the vaccine.

Experts were indeed worried; Dr Johnson State Public Health Officer in Michigan and a member of Advisory Committee on Immunisation Practises (ACIP) had this to say:

> *"This association leads me to favor a recommendation that infants up to two years old not be immunized with Thimerosal containing vaccines if suitable alternative preparations are available...*
>
> Dr Johnson

One of the main concerns seemed to be, how do the various health agencies manage the findings, how were they to break the news to the public, if at all, were they to keep the results secret until further studies were carried out? This was actually not an option as delegates knew the transcript of the meeting would soon be available to the public under the freedom of information act. What were lawyers acting on behalf of the vaccine damaged going to do with the results, how was this going to affect litigation against the drug companies?

> *"I know how we handle it from here is extremely problematic. So I leave you with the challenge that I am very concerned that this has gotten this far, and that having got this far, how you present in a concerted voice the information to the ACIP in a way they will be able to handle it and not get exposed to the traps which are out there in public relations.*
>
> *"I have the deepest respect for the work that has been done and the deepest respect for the analysis that has been done, but I wonder how on earth you are going to handle it from here."*

Dr Clements WHO

It was against this back drop that a further study was carried out that could <u>not</u> confirm the above, and at that very moment Dr Verstraeten the lead author of the study was effectively bought up from the CDC and employed by GlaxoSmithKline, a vaccine manufacturer of thimerosal–containing vaccines, a major pharmaceutical company presently facing a potentially large number of lawsuits on the very issue that the paper discusses.

Accusations of cover up, conflict of issues and impropriety ensued, which were of course vigorously denied. The follow-up study did not in fact confirm 'no link' as Dr Verstraeten himself acknowledges. In the furore to condemn the lack of confirmation, some critics had missed the point that the study was in fact neutral, there could still be a link, but the new study couldn't confirm it one way or the other.

*"The article does not state that we found evidence against an association, as a negative study would. It does state, on the contrary, that **additional study is recommended**, which is the conclusion to which a neutral study must come. Does a neutral outcome reduce the value of a study? It may make it less attractive to publishers and certainly to the press, but it in no way diminishes its scientific and public health merit. "*

Dr Verstraeten

There is of course a growing distrust of official reports and any evidence or suspicion of misconduct is seized upon by the vaccinated aggrieved in an attempt to receive some kind of justice. The reactions are understandable, yet as evidenced through the transcript it is apparent to me at least that all of those individuals representing the various organisations appear honest and industrious; they conduct experiments with integrity and are interested in safeguarding the health of the communities in their care.

By all accounts the actions of Dr Verstraeten seem flawless, he has acted with integrity both before his employment by GSK and since, finalising his involvement with the study before his departure from the CDC. How is it then possible to reconcile such conflicting views between those defending vaccines and those convinced of their harm?

One problem is that the scientists involved in those studies are constrained within very restrictive parameters, which makes their job immensely difficult. The study headed by Verstraeten was too see if only one component of certain vaccines, that are given to virtually everybody in the population, can cause certain kinds of neurodevelopmental disorders, conditions that take some time to develop and that can be potentially caused by many things.

Vaccines themselves contain all kinds of potentially harmful components, there are very few people to compare these studies to that are not vaccinated, practically an entire population is systematically vaccinated from a very young age and they are <u>not</u> systematically screened for adverse effects. Therefore scientists are only able to study the numbers of individuals whose parents report these conditions which are subsequently reported to the various health authorities.

In spite of all these limitations Dr Verstraeten was able to design a study that was able to demonstrate a relationship between thiomersal-containing vaccines and neurodevelopmental disorders but as ethical as he maybe, the fact remains that he was subsequently 'bought' by GlaxoSmithKline and consequently taken away from the CDC and away from the possibility of future studies on vaccine damage, to work for the very company facing litigation on that same issue. There was, on the face of it, no impropriety on his part but inevitably 'big pharma' can afford to 'buy out' the best scientists to conduct the experiments that they want, because you can rest assured that GSK will not be spending any sums of money repeating the kinds of studies that Dr Verstraeten conducted at the CDC.

The fault lies in the overall system, individual researchers are aware of the restrictions of their retrospective vaccine studies and do seem to do their level best to circumvent these limitations, but there is only so much they can achieve given their specific remit. They know that more definitive answers could be attained with properly controlled trials, but that is also considered unethical, they are of course partly blinded by their own faith in vaccines that considers the advantages of vaccines to outweigh the disadvantages.

> *I think the bottom line is that while the zero group is different, and I think all of us would agree with that, the issue is that it is impossible, unethical, to leave kids unimmunized, so you will never, ever resolve that issue. So then we have to refer back from that.*

> Dr Chen (Simpsonwood, June 2000)
> Chief of Vaccine Safety & Development at the
> National Immunization Program, CDC

They are also employed by health agencies that promote vaccination, consequently they have a duty to vaccinate and when looking at single pieces of evidence that could undermine public confidence in vaccines they want to be absolutely certain that it is true, which is entirely proper, but they are also influenced by the implications, a small problem with a vaccine could create a lack of public confidence in vaccines, its significance will be reduced if on balance they fear it could cause the rejection of a vaccine.

> *"My mandate as I sit here in this group is to make sure at the end of the day that 100,000,000 are immunized with DTP, Hepatitis B and if possible Hib, this year, next year and for many years to come..."*
>
> Dr Clements, WHO

The danger is that there are of course many findings across the spectrum of vaccine damage; singularly they may appear less significant and so singularly they are always glossed over as insignificant compared to the value of vaccination, but when added together they firmly tip the balance out of favour of vaccination.

But for many scientists the desire to safeguard a vaccine policy does not justify the rationale of waiting for more and more definitive proof, before applying caution. Dr. Boyd Haley, Chairman of the Chemistry Department at the University of Kentucky in correspondence with Mark Sircus Ac., O.M.D. Director International Medical Veritas Association indicated that the IOM is "blatantly out of line," and reduces the IOM report to the level of "absurd logic." He states:

> "The IOM report represents an incredibly poor evaluation of the scientific literature and is symptomatic of a committee that has been compromised in its scientific/biomedical credibility to favour the wishes of its employer, the CDC...Thimerosal is one of the most toxic compounds I know of, I can't think of anything that I know of is more lethal...I was amazed that the IOM would make such ridiculous statements and chose to use such

obviously damaged epidemiological studies to support their conclusions."

What is also very clear is that there is a complete double standard in vaccine policy; the great scientific minds that have been used to critically analyse evidence that vaccines are causing harm are not being used to investigate the evidence that vaccines are safe or effective; they are of course not the same thing. We are accepting vaccine safety and efficacy on very poor evidence unless proven dangerous, whereas it would be more appropriate to adopt the precautionary principle, accepting that they are harmful and ineffective unless proven to be safe and effective. If we used the same amount of intelligent and honest enquiry in assessing vaccine safety and effectiveness as we do in assessing the legitimacy of the evidence of harm, then vaccines would never make it into public health policy in their present form.

Vaccine promoters use the declining incidence of disease in populations as evidence of vaccine efficacy when clearly the majority of decline happens as a result of other factors. Even declines in disease incidence over and above what would be expected from vaccines are quick to be assigned as a consequence of the vaccination 'herd effect' or other 'unknown' non-specific effects. To accept vaccine damage, evidence undergoes the most rigorous scientific examination, to accept vaccine effectiveness evidence is almost whimsical.

For example diphtheria vaccine can at best only stimulate antibodies to the toxin produced by the bacteria and studies show that this does not change the number of people that contract diphtheria.

It is presumed that this vaccine can at best reduce the severity of the disease, but because the actual incidence of the disease has dropped over the years, intelligent, honest and reliable researchers will blindly state that this must be due to some effect of the vaccine, as though no other factors could influence disease rates, humans really are presumed to have no protection against disease unless vaccinated.

"However, If diphtheria toxoid vaccines did not impart any protection against infection, then one might predict that there should have been no change in the incidence of C. diphtheriae infection in the community and no change in the risk of disease in unvaccinated individuals."

Paul E.M. Fine Epidemiologic Reviews 1993 Johns Hopkins University, Vol. 15, No. 2

To reiterate the above, the researcher Paul Fine believes that if the vaccine doesn't reduce diphtheria infection then there would be no change in the incidence of diphtheria, the assumption is diphtheria rates can't possibly go down unless the vaccine is doing it. Of course all experience tells us that there are many factors of nutrition, sanitation, emotions and lifestyle that have influence on both the incidence and severity of all illnesses.

In addition, the initial vaccine toxicological studies are carried out on healthy people and therefore underestimate their impact on people with underlying health issues; this is then compared to the serious adverse events that can happen when some people contract a disease which only happens to those that already have an underlying illness. That is, millions of people may get measles but only the seriously immune compromised may suffer long-term damage, so in comparing the risks of vaccines (assessed by conducting trials on very few healthy adults) to the risks of illness, we are comparing vaccines in healthy to the consequences of the natural disease in the very sick.

When we are given the risks associated with a vaccine, that risk, only applies to vaccines in healthy people, which is therefore an underestimate of its true risk in the real population. We are then given the risks of the disease, which is in fact a statistic that differs from community to community and includes the very sick and immune compromised. This 'risk' will of course be completely inappropriate to everyone else. If the only people to suffer adverse effects of measles are in fact the seriously immune compromised, the risk of serious adverse effects to measles in somebody without that susceptibility is zero, however, the risk card is being played as a marketing tool used by the pharmaceutical industry, which is both misleading and unethical.

And so all of the various institutions, offices and laboratories around the world, are assessing individual issues with regard to vaccine dangers and each of them naturally assumes that their specific issue cannot counterbalance the benefit of vaccination and therefore underplays the relative importance of that issue.

But just as we do not assess the combination of toxic components within a vaccine, we assess mercury toxicity independently of aluminium toxicity when together the impact could be greater that the sum of the parts, likewise all of the various vaccine dangers are taken separately and nobody is joining up the dots, which is of course reflective of a medical perspective that similarly isolates the body into parts. The whole-body perspective is missing just as the whole vaccine perspective is missing and the dominant mantra of those supporting vaccines is the belief that the benefit of vaccines must outweigh the disadvantages. But what would be the impact of joining up the dots, collecting the relevant evidence irrespective of the consequence to our vaccine policy; would the advantages still outweigh the disadvantages?

So it is with regard to this specific thiomersal issue we are being told that the evidence is still not conclusive, so carry on vaccinating with thiomersal. But what would the experts do with their own children?

The results of the Verstraeten study into thimerosal and neurodevelopmental disorders presented at the Simpsonwood meeting were given on 'day one' of a two-day conference. On the morning of the second day Dr Johnson - State Public Health Officer in Michigan and a member of Advisory Committee on Immunisation Practises (ACIP) had this to say:

> *"Forgive this personal comment, but I got called out at eight o'clock for an emergency call and my daughter-in-law delivered*

a son by C-section. Our first male in the line of the next generation, and I do not want that grandson to get a Thimerosal-containing vaccine until we know better what is going on. It will probably take a long time. In the meantime, and I know there are probably implications for this internationally, but in the meanwhile I think I want that grandson to only be given Thimerosal-free vaccines"

As individuals with freedom of choice and sufficient evidence we naturally take the precautionary principle, many individuals looking at the issue of vaccination are in fact doing just that, they are not 'un-protecting' themselves they are betting on 'natural immunity'. We now have considerably more individuals opting out of one or other vaccine and in fact many opting out of all vaccines, we currently have large enough groups of individuals to compare vaccinated against non-vaccinated. Such comparative studies are not completely without bias because the unvaccinated group are self selected and may have alternative strategies of health care, however many of those factors are far easier to accommodate than previous studies where we have virtually no comparison group. So what would be the results of such studies with real unvaccinated control groups and are the health authorities willing to conduct such studies and really put the value of vaccination on the line?

Much of the effort and rationale to vaccinating comes from a belief in the way the human body functions in health and disease, and how we contract infectious disease. However if we were to understand things differently; include the orthodox view within a bigger picture, we may be able to see things that are obscured when preoccupied with the detail. We shall now look at the human body in a more holistic manner than we commonly do in a strictly orthodox medical culture, to see if there are additional perspectives that can be added to our models of health, immunity and infectious illnesses.

CHAPTER TEN

10 How vaccines start a chain reaction of symptoms, drug escalation and serious illness.

"If the only tool you have is a hammer, you tend to see every problem as a nail."

Abraham Maslow

By vaccinating we are in fact injecting a potentially dangerous cocktail of poisons and possible pathogens into the body, and from what we know of our immune system, we would therefore expect an immune reaction; a reaction designed to minimise the progress of these elements further into the body, eliminate these elements entirely from the body, and ideally have learnt from the whole process such that we are now less susceptible to such a natural illness in the future.

The fact is, some individuals do respond with such immune reactions with symptoms of fever, possibly eliminative rashes and mucus production; however, these individuals are then strongly advised, by the same medical advisors administering the vaccines, to **suppress these immune reactions**. Suppress, using pharmaceutical medication such as calpol etc.

So, having injected dangerous poisons into the body in order to stimulate an immune response, any reactions designed to resolve the trauma (other than the internal production of antibodies) are then suppressed.

Vaccine promoters must therefore be saying that the blood immune response to vaccine poisons i.e. the production of antibodies, is ok, but any other associated response is not ok and should therefore be suppressed with medication. This is obviously an illogical and in fact very dangerous policy; especially in view of the fact that we **know** how vitally important reactions such as the generalised inflammatory response is, with subsequent rash and toxin elimination, and we don't know how exactly the immune system mounts an effective response to, for example, viruses. Therefore how can one rationalise suppressing aspects of our response, especially those aspects that we **know** are vitally important.

This point cannot be overstated; the whole purpose of vaccination is to stimulate the immune system, yet this is exactly what is being <u>suppressed</u> by the routine use of antipyretic and anti-inflammatory medication such as calpol or paracetamol after vaccination.

10.1 The problems persist

By the process of vaccination we are aware that vaccine elements are injected into the blood, which therefore bypasses most of the immune system; often there are no apparent attempts to eliminate these toxins. The body has been effectively tricked into accepting a vast array of toxins that ordinarily it does its utmost to keep out. Then, if there are any reactions, these are routinely suppressed with medication.

If these vaccine elements remain within the system, then not only do we have the problem of the effect of those poisons and immune complexes in the internal system, but we also have the problems inherent in the issue of **'unresolved'** elimination. We know that <u>unresolved</u> reactions lead to persistent similar reactions, that is to say,

...Acute reactions that are unsuccessful give rise to persistent chronic reactions.

This phenomenon is more fully explained in the follow-up book *'SomaWisdom – The Science of Health & Healing'* by Trevor Gunn

What are the possible implications of this with regard to vaccines?

The natural reaction to poisons taken into the blood would be a generalised inflammatory reaction involving dilation (widening) of blood vessels - bringing blood including the white blood cells to the affected area; plus increased permeability (leakiness) of the blood vessel wall and external membranes –allowing waste materials and white blood cells out.

This is a purposeful, sophisticated and coordinated response designed to enhance white blood cell destruction of toxins and microbes, with the elimination of waste matter across the membranes of the body. An injection of toxins into the blood from a vaccine that could **not** be eliminated via an acute elimination reaction (i.e. an elimination that would happen in a natural acute disease such as measles) could therefore lead to persistent chronic reactions.

Therefore could vaccination give rise to persistent low-level immune reaction including membrane leaking?

This has in fact been demonstrated and reported by Henry Pabst in the case of MMR vaccination and reported in Vaccine Vol. 15, issue 1, pages 10-14, titled "Kinetics of immunological responses after primary MMR vaccine" demonstrating the persistent presence of immune chemicals such as interferon gamma which has been demonstrated to cause an increased permeability of the membranes of the digestive tract and blood brain barrier. Thus the biological effects of vaccination on the membranes of those vaccinated have been demonstrated, illustrating the nature of the **unresolved** immune reaction that can happen as a consequence of vaccination. In such cases there has been no immune learning, but in fact immune failure.

From what we have discussed of the principles of "learning", an effective immune response, especially those that have been classified as the childhood illnesses, when **resolved,** gives rise to the successful elimination of toxins and microbes and a decreased susceptibility to ingested toxins. The systems become stronger, the membrane becomes **stronger,** (not weaker, i.e. not persistently more permeable as has been demonstrated with vaccines), after the resolution of natural illness we are less susceptible to allowing in other toxins and microbes from our food and environment.

Therefore the blood elimination reaction need only occur enough times to sufficiently strengthen the membranes and associated systems. Consequently we do not need to subject our **blood** to all possible environmental toxins in order to develop antibodies to each and every one of them, what vaccine producers consider to be 'immunity'.

Vaccinators do not understand the nature of immune learning, like any learning process, you do not need to be subjected to every possible problem to learn how to resolve them. When learning to ride a bike it is not necessary to bruise every surface of the skin or break every possible limb in the learning process. Similarly once you've mastered a right turn, then that's it, you are not going to fall over at every other different right turn you encounter. Similarly once you've learnt a specific toxin and microbe elimination, the nature of immune learning is such that the membrane has the ability to keep out all kinds of other toxins more efficiently than before the learning process.

Individuals with high levels of health that exist from year to year **without** symptoms of colds and flu **do not** have antibodies to all the different viruses and bacteria that are supposedly implicated in these diseases. Their external immune defences function sufficiently well to keep the necessary elements out of their blood system. That is the goal of a fully functional and developed immune system. Note, therefore, with vaccines the opposite has been demonstrated, vaccination injects toxins that are not eliminated from the blood system, creating membranes that are persistently leaky which would therefore lead to **increased susceptibility** to blood toxicity, and an increase in chronic immune reactions.

Far from becoming immune to the vaccine elements, in such instances individuals become **sensitised** to these elements with the added pathology of poor membrane function. Not only do they respond persistently to an ongoing problem but also the nature of the leaky membrane is such that they now allow in a wider range of foods, toxins and microbes. They become more susceptible to such pathogens entering their blood and from the vaccinators frame of reference they have every reason to develop even more vaccines in an attempt to address susceptibility to an infinite possibility of microbes and toxins. This is good news from a commercial point of view for those in the vaccine industry, but bad news for your immune system.

Is there any evidence of this when comparing actual disease rates in vaccinated and non-vaccinated individuals? On June 29, 1996 the Lancet reported on medical studies showing that children with a history of natural illnesses such as measles, mumps and rubella were less likely to suffer with **allergies** in later life. Researchers from Southampton General Hospital in the UK now confirm this, discovering that:

> *Children with a history of measles suffer less from allergic conditions such as asthma, eczema and hay fever when compared to vaccinated individuals.*

Similarly research by Michel Odent reported in the Journal of the American Medical Association (1994; 272:592-3) showed that the use of whooping cough vaccine increased the incidence of asthma by 5-6 times as compared to non-vaccinated children. This was later confirmed by research at Churchill Hospital in Oxford UK and presented to the British Thoracic Society by Chest Consultant, Dr Julian Hopkin.

If toxins have crossed the membranes of the body and have failed to be eliminated then the individual becomes <u>sensitised</u> to those substances and then has to develop new strategies to prevent any more of those substances entering the body and causing further problems.

10.2 More 'invasive' consequences

An accumulation of toxins beyond the blood and into the internal tissues of the body will be stored out of harms way in the connective tissue, fat deposits and the joints. Toxins will also collect in the liver where the body attempts most of the detoxification reactions. Toxins and immune complexes will also collect by default in the kidneys where the fine capillaries filter out waste into the urine, and occasionally at the heart valves. Consequently these are the most common places where acute and chronic immune reactions occur. Here we see acute and chronic symptoms of cellulites, arthritis, nephritis, hepatitis and rheumatic heart disease.

The body has been doing its best to eliminate toxins, microbes and cellular debris from its interior thereby protecting the internal tissues of the body, and it is especially **important to protect** the cells of the **nervous system**.

When poisons, waste, cell debris and microbes build around the nerve cells, the failure of acute and chronic symptoms here could lead to neurological problems resulting in long-term damage, including paralysis, loss of sensory function, brain damage and even death. In the acute we see illnesses such as acute flaccid paralysis and infantile paralysis (*later called paralytic poliomyelitis in an attempt to attribute the pathology to the polio virus*), meningitis, encephalitis, and the chronic illnesses such as autism, attention deficiency syndromes, ME, Alzheimer's and so on. These are the invasive illnesses that the body is doing its utmost to avoid, but in fact most suppressive medication, including vaccines, actually predisposes us to.

10.3 Waning vaccine immunity

With the vaccine community promoting the idea that vaccines create immunity, they have to reconcile the fact that this so-called immunity is not life long as is natural immunity. We are therefore told that vaccine immunity wears off, which of course requires that we are given repeat doses of the vaccine. If we understand the nature of immune development and acknowledge the integration of our physiological systems together with mind and body we realise that immune development and consequently immunity, like learning to do anything, walking talking, eating etc, **cannot wear off**.

The only possibility of un-learning something is if we deteriorate so markedly in health that we become susceptible to ill-health generally, as is often the case in elderly, mal-nourished, severely traumatised etc. There can be no specific un-learning of one disease, **the reason vaccine immunity appears to wear off is that there was no immune learning in the first place,** immunity has merely been delayed. With or without antibodies vaccinated individuals will succumb to those illnesses in the future if the issues of susceptibility come up later. Childhood illnesses occur later because the individual has had to overcome deeper problems before they could be healthy enough to express the childhood illness; these deeper problems are often exacerbated by the vaccine.

If a child has been forced to stop crying whilst experiencing an upset, then at some point in the future this upset may be expressed. The expression was however suppressed and the child has had to deal with the additional trauma of being made to feel wrong, bad, unsupported etc. If fortunate the child may eventually get to express the original upset, at this point there is no un-learning of any ability to deal with the trauma, it was never dealt with in the first place.

>**Rather than creating a waning immunity, vaccines <u>delay</u> immunity.**

With sufficient overview of the disease process, the effects of vaccines are predictable. If you read the packet inserts of vaccines, even the acknowledged adverse effects amount to a catalogue of potential biological disasters; the medical profession and vaccine producers know that harmful effects occur:

> ➢ *Redness, swelling, soreness or tenderness at the vaccine site, mild to moderate fever, tiredness, drowsiness, poor appetite, headache, nausea, vomiting, mild rash, seizure (jerking or staring), non-stop crying - for 3 hours or more, high fever, swelling of the lymph nodes (lymphadenopathy), inflammation of the parotid gland (a salivary gland near the ear), low platelet count (thrombocytopenia) which can cause a bleeding disorder, serious allergic reaction (breathing difficulty, shock), pneumonia, pain and stiffness in the joints (mostly in teenage or adult women), chronic and acute arthritis, nerve inflammation, long-term seizures, severe paralytic illness (Guillain-Barré Syndrome), coma, or lowered consciousness, brain inflammation (encephalitis), permanent brain damage and death.*

The main problem of vaccine promoters is that they do not understand how, why and in what percentage of individuals these reactions occur. A situation not helped by the fact that adverse reporting is known to be a fraction of the true figure. As noted in the preceding text, the under-reporting of drug side-effects is a world-wide phenomenon:

> *In total, 37 studies using a wide variety of surveillance methods were identified from 12 countries. These generated 43 numerical estimates of under-reporting. The median **under-reporting rate** across the 37 studies **was 94%.***

> L.Hazell & S.A Shakir, International journal of toxicology
> Drug safety 2006; 29(5):385-96

CHAPTER ELEVEN

11 Why vaccines in some people are a 'Fast-Track' to serious disease.

The human body is designed to:

> ➤ Provide effective barriers to invasive poisons and microbes.
> ➤ Eliminate toxins accumulated from within.
> ➤ Limit the effects of toxins that have not been eliminated.

Vaccines can in one single instance bypass those systems, poisoning the internal tissues and nervous system, potentially creating illnesses that would ordinarily take many years of immune failure and/or extreme poisoning to produce.

11.1 Polio vaccine

Paralytic poliomyelitis is one such invasive illness, involving inflammation of the nervous system including the brain. The term paralytic poliomyelitis was a term used to describe what was previously described as acute flaccid paralysis or infantile paralysis.

Dr Morton S. Biskind's published articles in 1953 illustrates that the epidemics of the 50's and 60's have in fact been clearly linked to the use of the insecticides DDT (Dichlorodiphenyltrichloroethane), BHC (benzene haxachloride), Arsenic and Lead insecticide compounds, produced by the agrochemical industry, they were also components of household fly killer produced at the same time. These insecticides inevitably found their way into our food and being potent neurological poisons, caused acute neurological poisoning, paralysis, long-term weakness, muscle wasting, brain damage and even death in susceptible individuals.

Jim West's article 'Images of Poliomyelitis - A Critique of Scientific Literature' illustrates the close correlation between the use of these pesticides and the increase in cases of paralytic diseases. Many pharmaceutical researchers were however far more inclined to search for an offending microbe thereby following the pattern that had been reinforced years earlier with Pasteur. The orthodox medical profession would ignore issues of susceptibility, ignore individual environmental and or lifestyle issues, ignore the impact of commercial farming and industrialised pollutants in their attempts to understand and combat disease.

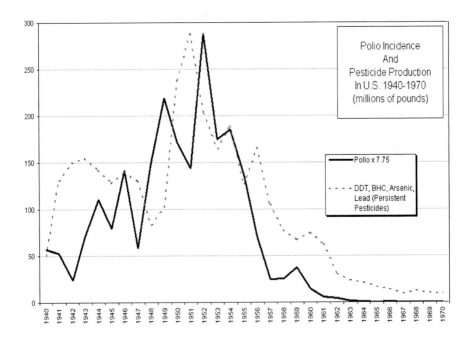

Jim West quotes from Biskind's 1953 article published in the 'American Journal of Digestive Diseases.'

"In 1945, against the advice of investigators who had studied the pharmacology of the compound and found it dangerous for all forms of life, DDT (chlorophenoethane, dichlorodiphenyl-trichloroethane) was released in the United States and other countries for general use by the public as an insecticide. Since the last war there have been a number of curious changes in the incidence of certain ailments and the development of new syndromes never before observed. A most significant feature of this situation is that both man and all his domestic animals have simultaneously been affected. "

"It was even known by 1945 that DDT is stored in the body fat of mammals and appears in the milk. With this foreknowledge the series of catastrophic events that followed the most intensive campaign of mass poisoning in known human history, should not have surprised the experts."

The polio virus was found at the site of the nerve damage and has been promoted as *'the cause'* of polio for many years, even though researchers at the time insisted this was not an infectious disease but a neurological poisoning. However, various vaccines were produced with questionable effects in an attempt to cash in on a drug-based preventative.

The reduction of polio however coincided with the banning of DDT and other compounds in the 1970's. However, where they are still in use today in developing countries for example in Nigeria there are once again high rates of infantile paralysis (polio by another name).

11.1.1 Problems with the polio virus theory:

➢ These viruses are found naturally in the digestive system of most individuals, therefore there would need to be a trigger to enable these to either, enter the blood and gain access to the nerves, or another trigger (such as a neurological poison) that would enable the formation of such viruses at the site of nerve damage. Remember it has been shown that viruses are created when we poison cells.

> To date there are at least 72 viruses of the same family of the original polio viruses that can also be found at the site of neurological damage in syndromes that are identical to paralytic poliomyelitis. We vaccinate against only three of these 72 viruses

> In many instances of illnesses that are clinically indistinguishable from paralytic poliomyelitis, polioviruses are not present. We therefore have acute paralytic diseases that have been renamed according to the presence of these other viruses, e.g. coxsackie viral paralysis, and echo viral paralysis. (The Lancet, 1962:548-51).

> The chronic symptoms of polio that remain in cases that do not completely resolve is called post-polio syndrome, separate syndromes have also been classified according to other viruses of the polio family and these syndromes have since been reclassified under the general headings of 'post viral syndrome', 'ME' and more recently 'chronic fatigue syndrome'.

> Isolation of the virus from affected victims is in fact a mixture of cell debris and toxins from the damaged tissue, this, needs to be injected into the brains of animals in order to create symptoms of paralysis. Polio, however, is never caused by injections into the brain.

Neurological poisoning in such acute and chronic syndromes is in fact due to many factors of which vaccines have been shown to contribute, rather than prevent. There are in fact dozens of studies that have appeared in orthodox research journals showing the link between vaccines (and other injections) and the onset of paralytic poliomyelitis. As early as 1900's, the early vaccines of diphtheria and whooping cough were known to induce paralysis with the paralysis starting in the vaccinated limb.

HV Wyatt has presented evidence in the *'Bulletin of Historical Medicine'* 1981; 55:543-57 showing that many kinds of injections could precipitate paralytic poliomyelitis. He has also shown that paralysis starting in both sides of the body is in fact prevalent in individuals receiving injections on both sides. Unfortunately the WHO diagnoses such cases as Guilaine Barre Syndrome as it has been decided that paralytic poliomyelitis appears on one side of the body only.

> According to Sir Graham S Wilson, honorary lecturer at the Department of Bacteriology, London School of Hygiene and Tropical Medicine, many different types of **vaccine can precipitate polio** (GS Wilson, The Hazards of Immunization, 1967:265-80).

> In 1992 RW Sutter studying a large outbreak of paralytic poliomyelitis in Oman, published a report in the Journal of Infectious Diseases showing that children who received DPT (diphtheria, tetanus, and pertussis) injections were more likely than controls to suffer paralytic poliomyelitis within the next 30 days, concluding that **"injections are an important cause of provocative poliomyelitis"**

> PM Strebel reported in The New England Journal of Medicine in 1995 that children who received a single intramuscular injection within one month after receiving a polio vaccine were **8** times more likely to contract polio than children who received no injections, when children received up to nine injections within one month they were **27** times more likely to contract polio and a staggering **182** times more likely to contract polio with ten or more injections.

Through the minutia of viral disease classification, vaccine producers have managed to give the impression that infantile paralysis and acute flaccid paralysis was caused by a virus, rather than a neurological poisoning from the insecticide industry. Vaccine promoters have then tried to say, that as a result of vaccination, polio has declined and that post-polio syndromes are rare. In fact such conditions as stated by the original researchers are neurological poisonings and vaccines have been clearly shown to contribute to the increase of these illnesses.

Inevitably there are questions that remain; some illnesses and consequently some vaccines appear to present unique scenarios that require specific attention. Polio, tetanus, and rubella for their own reasons seem to fall under that category, having looked at polio so we shall take some time to look at the tetanus and rubella vaccines in turn.

11.2 Tetanus

11.2.1 The vaccine appears to mimic the disease

This is an illness that is due to bacterial toxins from the site of a wound affecting the nervous system and therefore, unlike other illnesses, does appear to be more closely related to the process of vaccination. The tetanus bacteria themselves (Clostridium tetani) are widespread and can be found in soil, dust, manure, rust and even in the digestive tract of people. However, the issues are the same as other illnesses, firstly the symptoms of tetanus, paralysis and rigidity, are due to poisoning of the nervous system, often the first signs are in the jaw, hence the term lock-jaw. This nerve poisoning is in fact the end result of a disease process that can easily be avoided once we are clear about the causes.

If a wound contains enough material for bacteria to live on and is covered with no access to air, then the bacteria will grow without oxygen (anaerobically) this could give rise to the bacterial toxin that could lead to blood poisoning. Therefore shallow cuts and grazes do not pose such a problem and therefore in deeper injuries the first preventative is wound cleaning; this does not require topical antibacterial treatments as the presence of bacteria are not a problem, so long as the debris on which they live is removed. Thus wound cleansing has been recommended in Accident and Emergency departments utilizing tap water only, the Drugs and Therapeutics Bulletin of 25 November 1991 states that antibacterial applications actually slow wound healing making the situation worse, therefore tap water is recommended even in the A & E departments of hospitals.

11.2.2 Vaccines have no impact in most cases

Cases and mortality are higher in developing countries with poor hygienic conditions, here tetanus is significantly higher in newborns and most cases are caused by using dirty, rusty scissors when cutting the umbilical cord at birth in families that are poor and mal-nourished. Consequently these cases cannot be protected from vaccines since the vaccine is not given on the day of birth and cannot be effective in reducing the incidence of such conditions, therefore vaccines that are said to reduce tetanus in developing countries will actually have no impact on the majority of childhood tetanus cases.

11.2.3 Low vaccine rates – no tetanus

If, for example, a wound did contain debris, bacteria and no oxygen then the patient would experience a blood poisoning, in which case the site would become red and inflamed. Almost all patients in developed countries that are not specifically unwell with immune compromised conditions have an immune system and therefore would react successfully to such a wound. In fact tetanus is virtually unheard of in developed countries, vaccines, however, cannot be the reason for this, because it is estimated that at least 40% of these populations do not have up to date shots of tetanus. In the building industry where this figure may be higher and the nature of these wounds is a common everyday occurrence, there are no reported cases tetanus. Clearly natural immunity plays the most significant role in preventing this illness.

11.2.4 Tetanus a long process

If, therefore, a deep wound was not cleaned, there were sufficient bacteria and debris, the wound was covered allowing in no oxygen and the patient was unable to exhibit a successful inflammatory response, then blood poisoning could develop with concomitant symptoms. Even this can be treated, the wound can be surgically cleaned, the bacteria are sensitive to penicillin and there are many alternative treatments for this as well as effective nutritional advice that will help alleviate the problem. In such instances hospitals also use an antiserum sometimes called a passive vaccine containing antibodies to the toxin that are then supposed to alert your own white blood cells to the tetanus toxin within the blood and lymphatic system. But the body will still have the job of eliminating this poison from the system, there is also no guarantee that the body will not react to these foreign antibodies in the antiserum thus increasing the immune load as opposed to helping it.

If, however, a patient had a deep wound, that was covered, and the patient's immune response was so low that an inflammatory reaction could not deal with the wound, and or the inflammatory symptoms were suppressed and therefore this blood poisoning was not dealt with successfully, then the poison could become invasive and ultimately affect the nervous system.

So there are in fact a whole host of reactions and systems that come into play so that toxins from injuries do not become invasive and affect the nerves, this is actually what the body is designed to do, and continually does so from the moment of birth. The risk of this illness is more or less zero in the developed world, unless the individual is already immune compromised and likely to live in a situation where their injuries do not get basic care. The medical portrayal of tetanus gives the impression that the neurological consequences are likely, immediate and severe, from the smallest of cuts in any individual.

But of course the question still remains; will the vaccine help? Once again we are back to the main problems of all vaccines, the vaccine does not promote a full immune response, and should there be any reaction to the vaccine, i.e. inflammatory symptoms in response to the toxic burden of the vaccine contents, these symptoms will usually be suppressed by the very medical profession that administers the vaccine. The vaccine contents poison the system directly in the blood and therefore remain in the system adding to the immune burden in the short-term with possible long-term effects.

11.2.5 Tetanus vaccine - the real effects

Writing in the 'New England Journal of Medicine' 1984, 310(3): 198-199, Eibl et al reported that tests on 11 healthy adults before and after routine tetanus booster vaccines showed a significant though temporary drop in T- helper cell response (creating a high T-suppressor to T-helper activity) and significantly four of the eleven T-cell responses dropped to levels found in active AIDS patients and therefore research on the tetanus vaccine implicate vaccines as a cause of immune compromised reactions rather than enhanced immune responses. Dr Harold E. Buttram, M.D. has been in private medical practice since 1962, is board certified in Environmental Medicine, and Fellow of the American Academy of Environmental Medicine comments on the significance of these findings:

> *"If this was the result of a single vaccine in healthy adults, it is sobering to think of possible consequences from today's multiple vaccines routinely administered to infants. And yet, to the best of my knowledge, this study has never been repeated...*
>
> *... These studies do not constitute proof of harm from vaccines, but they are important clues. What they do prove is an ongoing pattern of negligence of many years in following up on these and other similar studies."*

Dr Kris Gaublomme, a medical doctor practising in Belgium researching the medical literature on tetanus vaccine also demonstrates the lack of scientific validity behind the use of the tetanus vaccine. Quoting research from Passen & Andersen, published in the Journal of the American Medical Association, (1988; 25519:1171-3):

> *"There is no absolute or universal protective level of antibody... The level of neutralizing antibody in humans currently considered protective, 0.01 antitoxin unit/ml, is based on animal studies that correlated levels with symptoms or death"*
> *Vieira, et al published in Med J Australia. 1986; 145: 156-7 confirm this: "This minimal protective level is an arbitrary one and is not a guarantee of security for the individual patient"...*

Other researchers have similarly found that high levels of antibodies to the contents of the vaccine do not protect against the toxins in the actual disease, Crone and Reder published research in 'Neurology' (1992; 42:761-4) describe a patient, in which the immunity to tetanus toxoid (in the vaccine) was not paralleled by immunity to tetanus neurotoxin (produced during the disease).

Dr Kris Gaublomme after reviewing the extensive medical literature on vaccine damage due to tetanus vaccine came to the following conclusion:

> *"The overwhelming amount of literature on tetanus toxoid vaccine adverse side-effects and the severity of those complications make it absolutely impossible to ridicule them as rare and benign. Doing so could only demonstrate a profound lack of knowledge of the literature concerned.*
>
> *Cunningham, Brindle and others insist on having adrenalin readily available when tetanus toxoid is administered, thus admitting that the vaccination is in fact a life-threatening medical intervention, even in apparently healthy individuals. This speaks for itself. Risking one's life by an intervention which is probably ineffective, to avoid a disease which will probably never occur is not sound medical practice. All it takes,*

on a world scale, to avoid the majority of tetanus cases is clean scissors to cut the newborn's umbilical cord. Information, soap and peroxide might do a far better job than tetanus vaccine."

As such the tetanus issue runs a parallel to all invasive consequences of any so-called infectious disease. All illnesses can become invasive, whether from the lungs, skin, digestive tract, or injuries etc, whatever the point of entry, the issue is the same, if the invasive toxins are not dealt with, then the consequences may eventually affect the nervous system and could lead to the death of the patient, this makes tetanus no different to any other infectious illness, whether it is measles, mumps, flu or polio, the vaccines, rather than help, add to the immune burden.

It is interesting to note that health authorities also recommend booster shots every 5-10 years because the so-called immunity wears off and currently in the UK within the National Health Service it is <u>only</u> possible to have a tetanus booster as a combination vaccine that would also containing diphtheria and pertusis, which raises the question; is there a biological justification for this or a commercial one?

Interestingly the only case of lockjaw I have ever treated was in a lady that had just received the tetanus vaccine for an injury where the bruising had not even broken the skin and where there was of course, no natural possibility of tetanus. Her symptoms were actually from the vaccine.

11.3 Rubella

11.3.1 Rubella vaccine - what's the point?

Rubella (German measles) presents an apparently different challenge; the disease itself is fairly mild in children and is associated with the rubella RNA virus that is assumed to be the cause of the disease and believed to be there if certain antibodies are detected in the blood. The condition presents as a mild inflammatory condition starting with tiredness, aching, fever and often swollen lymph glands on the neck, a red-pink rash appears 3-4 days after the first symptoms and last for around a week. The spots usually start behind the ears, before spreading around the head, neck, face, and after 2-3 days develop on the trunk and the extremities.

Complications arising from the childhood disease are similarly mild, rare and not cause for concern within the medical profession, the condition can be more severe if contracted in adulthood affecting the joints with pain, swelling and/or inflammation, there are also cases of thrombocytopenia, (reduced blood platelets – the cells involved in blood clotting).

However, if women contract the disease during pregnancy it can result in the birth of the child with multiple congenital deformities or lead to spontaneous abortion. The justification for the use of the vaccine is therefore for the safety of the unborn child, to protect the child from what is called 'congenital rubella syndrome' (CRS) and the concomitant devastating effects on the parents and the rest of the family, which is of course a noble goal; however, let's take a closer look at this issue.

11.3.2 Vaccine versus natural immunity

In determining the frequency of rubella and ultimately the effectiveness of a vaccine program it is important to realise that the diagnosis of rubella is not as straightforward as it appears. Firstly the symptoms of rubella could just appear as swollen glands and may not even show the rash at all. There could even be no symptoms at all and evidence of rubella virus, ascertained by the presence of certain antibodies; therefore sub-clinical infection (detected presence of antibodies but no symptoms of illness) is known to be very common.

With regard to assessing the effectiveness of the vaccine in terms of reducing the incidence of the disease, this again relies on reported cases of rubella, which is fraught with inaccuracies given that the symptoms often go unnoticed and can be mistaken for many illnesses diagnosed as non-specific viral rashes of childhood and often confused with measles and roseola.

> *"Despite detailed descriptions, however, exanthem subitum (roseola) tends to be confused with measles and rubella"*
>
> BMJ 312:101-102 (13 January 1996)

The initial concern with rubella vaccine (often given in the form of the measles, mumps and rubella triple vaccine MMR) is that rather than conferring lasting immunity it delays the onset of rubella from childhood to teenage and adult years, thus making the likelihood of contracting the illness in the child-bearing years even greater. The American Center for Disease Control thus reported in 1990:

> *"Before rubella vaccines became available in 1969, most rubella cases occurred among school-age children. Because control of rubella in the United States was originally based on interrupting transmission, the primary target group for vaccination was children of both sexes. Secondary emphasis was placed on vaccinating susceptible adolescents and young adults, especially females.*
>
> *By 1977, vaccination of children greater than or equal to 12 months of age had resulted in a marked decline in the reported rubella incidence among children and had interrupted the characteristic 6- to 9-year rubella epidemic cycle. However, this vaccination strategy had less effect on reported rubella incidence among persons greater than or equal to 15 years of age (i.e., the childbearing ages for women). This age group subsequently accounted for greater than 70% of reported rubella patients with known ages. Approximately 10%-20% of this latter population continued to be susceptible. **This proportion was similar to that of pre-vaccine years...**"*

> CDC Recommendations & Reports (23/11/1990) 39(RR15)

Therefore it was suggested that the vaccine hadn't impacted on the target group and that women of child-bearing age were just as likely to develop rubella since the introduction of the vaccine program. Some reports went further still, implying that the incidence in the target group was actually increasing since the use of rubella vaccine; Edward A. Mortimer Jr. MD et al in Pediatrics Vol. 65 No. 6 June 1980, pp. 1182-1184

> *"However, since the use of rubella vaccine has not been universal in the target population (only about two thirds of the children 1 to 12 years old have been immunized) and since vaccine usage has disrupted the epidemic nature of rubella, the population for whom antibody protection is desired **(women of childbearing age) is still suspected of being as susceptible, or more so, than in the pre-vaccine era.**"*

The natural illness carries minimal risk and would be far more effective at conferring natural immunity; it seems that the vaccine could be counterproductive in delaying natural immunity and creating a susceptibility to the illness at the worst time for women, during their child-bearing age. Robert S. Mendelsohn, M.D. in his book "The Medical Time Bomb of Immunization against Disease" is equally critical, quoting the efforts of other doctors to remove the vaccine from their mandated list.

> *"The greater danger of rubella vaccination is the possibility that it may deny expectant mothers the protection of natural immunity from the disease. By preventing rubella in childhood, immunization may actually increase the threat that women will contract rubella during their childbearing years. My concern on this score is shared by many doctors. In Connecticut a group of doctors, led by two eminent epidemiologists, have actually succeeded in getting rubella stricken from the list of legally required immunizations."*

11.3.3 Adverse effects – first do no harm

We therefore have a vaccine of questionable benefit, but we also have to look at this against the added risk of the vaccine in causing adverse effects. Adverse effects which are of course under-reported, as vaccine recipients are not routinely screened for potential vaccine reactions. However, when separate and independent research is conducted into the specific short and long-term effects of rubella vaccines (after the vaccine has been accepted in public health policy), many adverse reactions are found. There are numerous resources that list published research of the adverse effects of vaccines, one such resource is "Think Twice Global Vaccine Institute" found at www.thinktwice.com, and lists a simple, though not exhaustive list of such research, as follows:

> **The Rubella Vaccine and Arthritis:**
> Cooper, L.Z., et al. "Transient arthritis after rubella vaccination."
> *Am J Dis Child* 1969; 118:218-225.
> Spruance, S.L., et al. "Joint complications associated with derivatives of HPV-77 rubella virus vaccine." *American Journal of Diseases in Children* 1971; 122:105-111.
> Swartz, T.A., et al. "Clinical manifestations, according to age, among females given HPV-77 duck rubella vaccine." *American Journal of Epidemiology* 1971; 94:246-51.
> Weibel, R.E., et al. "Influence of age on clinical response to HPV-77 duck rubella vaccine." *J. of American Medical Association* 1972; 222:805-807.
> Thompson, G.R., et al. "Intermittent arthritis following rubella vaccination: a three year follow-up." *American Journal of Diseases of Children* 1973; 125:526-530.
> Chantler, J.K., et al. "Persistent rubella infection and rubella-associated arthritis." *Lancet* (June 12, 1982):1323-1325.
> Tingle, A.J., et al. "Prolonged arthritis, viraemia, hypogamma-globulinaemia, and failed seroconversion following rubella immunisation." *Lancet* 1984; 1:1475-1476.

Tingle, A.J., et al. "Postpartum rubella immunization: association with development of prolonged arthritis, neurological sequelae, and chronic rubella viremia." *Journal of Infectious Diseases* 1985; 152:606-612.

Tingle, A.J., et al. "Rubella-associated arthritis. Comparative study of joint manifestations associated with natural rubella infection and RA 27/3 rubella immunisation." *Annals of the Rheumatic Diseases* 1986; 45:110-114.

Institute of Medicine. *Adverse Effects of Pertussis and Rubella Vaccines.* (Washington, DC: National Academy Press, 1991).

Benjamin, C.M., et al. "Joint and limb symptoms in children after immunisation with measles, mumps, and rubella vaccine." *British Medical Journal* 1992; 304:1075-78.

The Rubella Vaccine and Neurological Disorders:

Kilroy, A.W., et al. "Two syndromes following rubella immunization." *Journal of the American Medical Association* 1970; 214:2287-2292.

Gilmarten, R.C., et al. "Rubella vaccine myeloradiculoneuritis." *Journal of Pediatrics* 1972; 80:406-412.

Schaffner, W., et al. "Polyneuropathy following rubella immunization: a follow-up study and review of the problem." *American Journal of Diseases of Children* 1974; 127:684-688.

Institute of Medicine. *Adverse Effects of Pertussis and Rubella Vaccines.* (Washington, DC: National Academy Press, 1991).

Muhlebach-Sponer, M., et al. "Intrathecal rubella antibodies in an adolescent with Guillain-Barre syndrome after mumps-measles-rubella vaccination." *European Journal of Pediatrics* 1994; 154:166.

Ehrengut, W. "Central nervous system sequelae of immunization against measles, mumps, rubella and poliomyelitis." *Acta Paediatrica Japonica* 1990; 32:8-11.

Aubrey, J., et al. "Postpartum rubella immunization: association with development of prolonged arthritis, neurological sequelae, and chronic rubella viremia." *Journal of Infectious Diseases* (September 1985); 152(3):606-612.

The Rubella Vaccine and Diabetes:

Menser, M., et al. "Rubella infection and diabetes mellitus." *Lancet* (January 14, 1978), pp. 57-60.

Rayfield, E.J., et al. "Rubella virus-induced diabetes in the hamster." *Diabetes* (December 1986); 35:1278-1281.

Coulter, Harris. "Childhood vaccinations and Juvenile-Onset (Type-1) diabetes." *Congressional Testimony. Committee on Appropriations, subcommittee on Labor, Health and Human Services, Education, and Related Agencies.* (April 16, 1997).

Coyle, P.K., et al. "Rubella-specific immune complexes after congenital infection and vaccination." *Infection and Immunity* (May 1982); 36(2):498-503.

Numazaki, K., et al. "Infection of cultured human fetal pancreatic islet cells by rubella virus." *American Journal of Clinical Pathology* 1989; 91:446-451.

The Rubella Vaccine and Chronic Fatigue Syndrome:

Tobi, M., et al. "Prolonged atypical illness associated with serological evidence of persistent Epstein-Barr virus infection." *Lancet* 1982; 1:61-64.

Bicker, U. "Some new aspects of autoimmunity." *Journal of Immuno-pharmacology* 1986; 8:543-559.

Allen, A.D. "Is RA27/3 rubella immunization a cause of Chronic Fatigue?" *Medical Hypotheses* 1988; 27:217-220.

Lieberman, A.D. "The role of the rubella virus in the chronic fatigue syndrome." *Clinical Ecology* 1991; 7(3):51-54.

Clearly adverse reactions do happen however numerous studies showing adverse events do not necessarily show whether the vaccine problems outweigh the benefits. But as we have previously discussed, legitimate controlled trials set up to assess benefit versus risk are not undertaken, therefore we can only make an informed guess as to benefit versus risk...but that guess equally applies to drug companies and health authorities in their faith in the vaccine; vaccine promoters 'guess' that the benefit outweighs the disadvantage.

11.3.4 Rubella vaccine - effective at doing what?

With regard to rubella vaccine effectiveness, most of the studies concentrate on the ability of the vaccine to produce antibodies in response to certain tests in the recipient, it seems it's easy to show that the vaccine can create an antibody response however would individuals develop sufficient antibodies naturally without vaccines? In 1982 the British Medical Journal 1,284, 628—30, reported on the antibody levels in rubella vaccinated 13 year old girls compared to boys that had not been vaccinated, showing that there was no statistically significant difference between vaccinated and non-vaccinated, you were as likely to produce antibodies naturally as you were with a vaccine.

However these tests do not focus on the actual incidence of rubella disease in these patients, i.e. these antibody trials do not tell us whether we are protected from contracting the actual disease or not, this is a point continually made by those criticising so-called vaccine 'evidence'. Viera Scheibner PhD in her book "Vaccination" quotes the report of Menser et al 'Impact of rubella vaccination in Australia' published in the Lancet 12/05/84.

> *After 13 years of rubella vaccination there has been a notable increase in the proportion of rubella sero-positive pregnant women (i.e. possessing anti-bodies). However, it is also true that 86% of a Melbourne ante-natal clinic's patients were sero-positive without any rubella vaccination.*

Viera Scheibner goes on to comment:

> *Without previous screening and testing and relating these data to **outbreaks of natural rubella**, these figures are really **meaningless**.*

Antibodies do not tell you whether you've been ill, are ill, or going to get ill, and therefore whether you are immune or not. To find studies addressing the most pertinent issue as to the disease rate of rubella in the vaccinated we have to go back to a time when researchers would have thought to question the role of vaccines, before the medical view became entrenched and oblivious to the need for such research.

Dr. Archie Kalokerinos qualified MD from Sydney University 1951, Medical Superintendent of Collarenebri Hospital until 1975. Fellow of the Royal Society for Health, International Academy of Preventive Medicine, Australasian College of Biomedical Scientists, Hong Kong Medical Technology Association, and New York Academy of Sciences. In 1978 he was awarded the A.M.M. (Australian Medal of Merit) for 'outstanding scientific research'. He tells of the research of Dr Beverly Allan Published in Australian Nurses Journal "Does Rubella Vaccination Protect?"

> "In October, 1972 a seminar on rubella was held at the Department of Pathology, University Department, Austin Hospital in Melbourne, Australia. Dr. Beverly Allen, a medical virologist, gave overwhelming evidence against the effectiveness of the vaccine. So stunned was she with her investigations that it caused her, like a growing number of scientists, to question the whole area related to herd immunizations. Dr. Allen described two trials: the first trial concerned army recruits who were selected because of their lack of immunity as determined by blood tests. These men were given Cendevax, an attenuated rubella virus that is supposed to protect. They were then sent to a camp which usually has an annual epidemic of rubella. This occurred three to four months after they were vaccinated, and 80% of the so-called immune recruits became infected with rubella virus. A further trial shortly after this took place at an institution for mentally retarded people with similar effects. Additional disturbing evidence was sent to us by a Melbourne doctor who was in the United Kingdom at the time that Chief Health Officer Sir Henry Yellowlees, had released a press statement (February 26, 1976) informing doctors that, in spite of high vaccination figures, there had been no detectable reduction in the number of babies born with birth defects"

11.3.5 Protecting the unborn

However the main issue is whether rubella vaccine specifically reduces the incidence of congenital rubella syndrome (CRS) in the unborn child and in so doing does not of course replace or even increase the incidence of other birth defects, i.e. do the advantages of the vaccine outweigh the risks of the vaccine to the unborn child?

> *"There are two kinds of statistics: the kind you look up and the kind you make up"*
>
> Rex Stout

Again we have to make assessments based on figures of congenital rubella syndrome before and after vaccination because no studies comparing vaccinated and un-vaccinated were carried out, however figures of disease rates before vaccination are apt to be exaggerated. Clifford Miller Lawyer and graduate physicist writing in the 'BMJ letters' 1/06/05 responds to a previous claim:

> "*In the United States ...in 1964 there were approximately 12.5 million cases of rubella, as many as 11,000 fetal deaths, and approximately 20,000 cases of congenital rubella.*"

Miller notes that the rubella disease figures used by the medical profession constitute scare stories that "...are **shocking** because they are **impossible**" he goes on to state:

> "*The authority cited was a 1984 article by, among others, Walter Orenstein, a Director of the US National Immunisation Programme. His job was to promote vaccination.*
>
> *The 1964 recorded rubella incidence for Maryland, USA, was, for example, 1:1000 population as reported Maryland Department of Health, 3,583 cases of rubella during 1964. (http://edcp.org/html/rubella.html accessed 30 May 2005). A*

*population of 3.9 million in 1970, increasing by 1/2 million every 10 years - provides estimated population 3.5 + million in 1964. The sub-group of CRS cases was typically 1:1000 of total rubella cases. The largest annual total of nationally reported cases of rubella in the United States was in 1969, when **57,681** cases were reported (58 cases per 100,000 population). At around **12,000 percent fewer** cases than the figures Mr Floyd cites.*

A web search produces numerous webpages repeating the figures Mr Floyd cites, referring to 1964 as a 'pandemic' and attributing the Orenstein paper as their source.

11.3.6 Congenital Rubella Syndrome (CRS)

More importantly however is the impact of rubella vaccine on congenital rubella syndrome (CRS), symptoms in the developing embryo that could lead to birth defects or death of the foetus. What exactly are the symptoms of CRS?

As with many illnesses there are two stages to consider; the immediate acute symptoms and if not resolved, the long-tem chronic condition. Steven Parker, MD at Boston University School of Medicine in his guide for parents and health professionals notes the conditions associated with what he terms early and delayed phases of CRS, observing that they also range from very mild to very severe:

*"Babies born with CRS are very different from each other. Some have significant disabilities, while others are barely affected. In fact, children with CRS are more likely to be different from each other than they are to be similar. **That's why it is difficult to present a typical picture of CRS. There is no typical picture."***

This of course makes it difficult if not impossible to assess the impact of a vaccine on a syndrome that varies widely in symptoms and in which the reporting of CRS has had no possibility of standardisation before and after the introduction of the vaccine. Unless a doctor decides to carry out their standard tests for rubella, it is highly likely that many individuals with these symptoms will not be diagnosed as having CRS.

According to Steven Parker, MD the acute early problems of CRS can be one or several of the following:

Hearing loss of any degree.

Vision problems ranging from normal to total blindness, problems include: Cataract (one or both eyes); inflammation of the retina (retinopathy); eye movement problems (nystagmus); and small eyes (microphthalmia); optic atrophy, corneal haze and glaucoma.

Heart problems which include: Patent ductus arteriosus; pulmonary artery stenosis, pulmonic valve stenosis; and ventricular septal defect.

Neurological problems or brain damage may or may not exist, may range from mild to very sever, problems can include: Small head (microcephaly); large soft spot of head (bulging fontanelle); lethargy; irritability; learning disabilities; mental retardation (mild, moderate, severe or profound); movement problems (cerebral palsy, spastic diplegia, hypotonia); poor balance and posture; lack of coordination; and seizure disorders.

Growth problems: Small size (intrauterine growth retardation).

Genitourinary Problems: Undescended testicles (cryptorchidism); hernia (inguinal hernia); hypospadias.

Other (Less Common) Problems: Swollen glands (adenopathy); liver inflammation (hepatitis); low blood count (hemolytic anemia); low platelet count (thrombocytopenic purpura); pneumonia (interstitial pneumonitis); bone lesions (metaphyseal striations); abnormal palm creases.

The delayed-onset manifestations of CRS in the main, affect the hormonal system and the brain, they include:

Insulin Dependent Diabetes Mellitus

Overactive thyroid gland (hyperthyroidism) or an underactive thyroid gland (hypothyroidism).

Glaucoma: While glaucoma is infrequent in infants with acute CRS, it may show up at a later time, especially if cataract surgery has been performed. While most ocular findings are present at birth, there are cases of eye problems emerging later in life (e.g. detached retinas), especially if head banging or eye poking is present.

Change in Hearing Ability: Both hearing loss and hearing gains have been recorded after the first few years of life.

Neurological System and Behaviour CRS may be characterized by poorly understood changes in the neurological system. New onset or changes in seizure disorder, changes in tone, posture, coordination and strength. Changes in behaviour or new behaviours occasionally develop over time including attention deficit disorder, impulsivity; self-injurious behaviours and **autistic** behaviours.

The impact of Rubella vaccine is therefore difficult enough to assess, but the assessment of the vaccine takes on a further twist when we consider that the evidence for the effectiveness of the vaccine is taken from the overall impression that we have fewer cases of birth defects since the use of the vaccine.

However routine abortion is offered to women that are suspected to have contracted rubella during pregnancy...

...which is of course a major factor influencing the numbers of birth defects presenting, add to that the various policies around the world of advising termination of pregnancies in foetuses with heart defects and other problems, we are of course eliminating the problems before they are born and have no way of assessing the impact of vaccines or any interventions in reducing birth defects by simply looking at the number of children born with these defects. They are bound to be lower since the introduction of routine abortion policies.

But the problems don't stop there, a cursory glance at our list of long term CRS symptoms may miss the fact that they also include:

> "...attention deficit disorder, impulsivity; self-injurious behaviours and **_autistic_** behaviours."

Are we to assume in this present climate that we have reduced the incidence of attention deficit disorders and autism? By extolling the virtues of rubella vaccine in reducing congenital disorders, how many people are aware that **autism** is part of the rubella syndrome that should of course be reducing as a result of vaccination, the main vaccine being MMR?

So again we have the typical vaccine scenario, evidence of antibody production used as evidence of the success of the vaccine without relating that to numbers of real disease cases, over exaggeration of the numbers of cases before the vaccine, no systemised screening for adverse effects of the vaccine, with many adverse effects found later but not used in an assessment of vaccine risk versus benefit and finally under-reporting of the disease in the vaccinated.

11.3.7 Controlled trials – unethical?

The definitive answers we are always told could be found by running prospective controlled trials, vaccinating half and compare to a non-vaccinated group, but the creation of a placebo (i.e. non-vaccinated) group is said to be unethical; unethical because we would be with-holding the vaccine from a group and thereby creating an avoidable risk of exposure to disease by with-holding a safe and effective vaccine. As discussed earlier, describing the creation of an unvaccinated group as being unethical presupposes that the vaccine is safer and more effective than natural immunity, which of course we do not know, unless we do the trials. This situation is even more questionable when we consider that many countries do not even use rubella vaccine. According to the Pan American Health Organization, (PAHO) Family and Community Health, immunization Unit, Washington, D.C. USA (a regional office of the World Health Organisation):

> "*... **42%** of the countries around the world that report to the World Health Organization (WHO) **still have not introduced rubella vaccine** into their national immunization programs.*"

Pan American Journal of Public Health 15(3), 2004

PAHO have therefore conducted various studies to determine if there is an '<u>unrecognised</u>' problem of CRS in one such country Haiti and therefore is there a case for introducing the vaccine in their public health program. An interesting use of resources considering the magnitude of their '**known**' health problems; according to a PAHO report "Health in the Americas 1998" commenting on conditions in Haiti:

> "*Water supply and basic sanitation services are still very deficient. No city has a public sewerage system...*
>
> *The leading causes of child mortality in Haiti are diarrheal diseases, acute respiratory infections, and malnutrition...*"

The health and social problems in Haiti are difficult to envisage for most people unaccustomed to such deprivation, the same report on Haiti elaborates:

> "*In 1991, the Center for Research on Human Resources conducted a survey in three cities in three different departments. The survey provided an overview of the plight of children (boys and girls under 18 years of age) in especially difficult circumstances, including several groups: children employed as domestics, abandoned children, orphans, incarcerated juvenile offenders, child prostitutes (male and*

female), abused children, and street children. The term "street children" refers to children whose only home is the streets and who only find food and shelter there. In 1991, the number of street children in Haiti ranged from 1,500 to 2,000 in Port-au-Prince,more than 100 in Le Cap Haïtien, and just under 100 in Les Cayes. Most of them are boys, but the number of girls appears to be increasing, accounting for 18% of the children surveyed in Port-au-Prince. The mean age of these children is about 11 years; 55% of them are aged 12 to 18 years old, and 14% are 5 years old or less. Their health problems include headaches, fatigue, insomnia, and anxiety. They are particularly vulnerable to tuberculosis, anemia, skin diseases, and sexually transmitted diseases. Many of these children are drug users (53% of the inner-city sample)."

Yet this regional office of the WHO feel justified in looking for other, as yet unrecognised problems in order to introduce more vaccinations, vaccines that they cannot afford, given their comment recognising: *"...the relatively high cost of the rubella vaccine for the average Haitian and the low socioeconomic status..."*

In spite of this, studies were conducted to provide estimates of rubella susceptible women finding that 95.2% were sero-positive and therefore as they conclude, leaving a relatively low group (4.8%) of susceptible individuals, their report states that:

"Even with an overall <u>low susceptibility</u> (seronegativity) rate of 4.8%, congenital rubella syndrome could still occur in Haiti."

Pan American Journal of Public Health Volume 15 (3) Mar 2004

So on the <u>possibility</u> of the syndrome occurring in only a small percentage of women further studies are conducted to assess the cost effectiveness of a mass rubella vaccination program. One such study reported in Pan American Journal of Public Health, Volume 12 (4), Oct 2002, tries to assess the possibility of this as yet unrecognised problem of CRS looking at *"three orphanages in Haiti that accept disabled children"*. They came to the conclusion that a probable 6 cases of CRS <u>may have occurred</u> and using data from USA prior to rubella vaccination and surrounding Caribbean countries they arrive at the conclusion that the rubella vaccine would be a cost-effective strategy in reducing the CRS disease burden of Haiti. PAHO are therefore promoting a vaccine to reduce an estimated disease burden that has so far been unrecognised, and even if real is completely dwarfed by the known health problems in Haiti, using a vaccine that they cannot afford which would inevitably remove resources from other areas of health care in a situation where they are desperately short of funds for even the most basic health provisions.

11.3.8 Ethical pharmaceuticals?

There does appear to be an issue of ethics in the promotion of vaccines under these circumstances, the avoidance of placebo controlled trials for 'ethical' reasons in countries where the vaccine is not used is a pharmaceutical ploy to drastically reduce the level of analysis of their vaccines. It would in fact be far simpler to conduct a prospective trial to really assess the worth of rubella vaccine, one would not be introducing a 'non-vaccinated' group; one would be introducing a vaccinated group and therefore be making assessments of the value of the vaccine against comparable controls i.e. against non-vaccinated individuals with natural immunity. In fact there are many opportunities world wide to conduct such studies, these studies would put to rest the criticisms of vaccines and address the issues of non-compliance in people that continually question the value of vaccines. These countries provide a genuine opportunity for vaccinators to demonstrate the real value of vaccines. Yet these organisations still persist in using worthless estimates of antibody levels, extrapolating data from other geographical areas to estimate possible disease rates, using no controls to assess the impact of the vaccine on actual disease rates, ignore confounding factors for example pregnancy terminations and conduct no health screening of vaccinated individuals when assessing vaccine safety once the vaccine is introduced into the population.

Individual health professionals and members of the public are then left to prove beyond a shadow of doubt whether a vaccine is safe or effective and therefore could on balance create more problems than it is solving. Whereas vaccine promoters use sloppy non-science to introduce a vaccine into public health policy without the need for proper studies, shielded by the circular reasoning of their 'ethical' argument for not conducting studies with proper controls.

We have looked at two specific examples, tetanus and rubella vaccines that often appear to present different challenges; however, as we can see, it is the same story in slightly different clothing as it is for all vaccines.

CHAPTER TWELVE

12 Do we really need to live in fear of dangerous viruses and the next pandemic?

12.1 Spanish Flu

Much of the impetus to the current measures to combat current illnesses for example, Bird Flu, Sars and Swine Flu etc comes from scientists' fear of a recurrence of an outbreak of disease similar to the 1918 Spanish Flu. An epidemic is an illness prevalent at one particular time affecting a national area. A pandemic affects large populations of the world at one time and the 1918 flu was a severe pandemic with a large death toll said to be due to a flu virus rampaging throughout much of Europe and eventually across the rest of the world.

In reality there were numerous reasons why the flu of the 1918 winter would have been more severe than any other. Firstly we were at the end of the First World War with a massive death toll, family bereavement and separation, appalling living conditions, malnutrition and unprecedented levels of fear.

Patients suffered from dehydration which would have been enough to kill them during any illness accompanied by a fever. Doctors were brought out of retirement to cope with illnesses because so many younger doctors were involved in the war, these replacement doctors would have been trained in the 1880's and were using very old and ineffective treatment methods. Reports show many patients had symptoms of aspirin overdose and side-effects from experimental vaccines and anti-sera.

Drugs may be responsible for many Flu pandemic deaths

Dr Karen Starko has re-examined autopsy reports from the 1918 flu and has found that many were consistent with aspirin toxicity and has come to the conclusion that high aspirin use could account for many of the 40 million deaths attributed to the flu virus.

> *Doctors were over-prescribing aspirin as they wanted to be doing something and yet they knew little about the drug's dangers, especially when taken at high doses. Under pressure to do something by families who were insistent on medical help, in addition the manufacturers were promoting aspirin use during the pandemic.* ***"Interventions cut both ways, "***

Dr Karen Starko,
Clinical Infectious Diseases, September 29, 2009

People were also displaying many different kinds of symptoms and these illnesses were given various disease names, eventually they grouped all of those illnesses together as Spanish Flu, but the symptoms were in no way consistent. It is only in retrospect that researchers are guesstimating that this could have been a viral illness, we have to remember that in 1918 there was no possibility of isolating and classifying viruses, the so-called 1918 Spanish Flu virus is a completely hypothetical virus.

Recent attempts to classify the 1918 flu virus have come from isolating pieces of genetic information (not actually isolating the virus) from a body that was approximately 90 years old; a diseased body that would have been filled with all kinds of dead cells, contaminant microbes and fragments of DNA. Then with the aid of laboratory techniques and computer simulation some scientists have tried to predict what the viral DNA and therefore what the microscopic virus would have been like that was responsible for millions of deaths in 1918.

The 1918 Spanish Flu that some vaccine promoters are saying could return if a virulent virus attacked, could <u>only</u> happen if the world's population descended into a scenario similar to the living conditions prevalent in 1918. The death toll was entirely related to the susceptibility of the individuals living at the end of the First World War and not due to a particularly virulent virus that wanted to kill as many people as possible. The fear of a repeat of the 1918 flu pandemic is borne out of a medical perception that perceives disease as something that has nothing to do with the patient, their susceptibility or their living conditions.

Neither was the high death toll due to a novel virus that we had no prior immunity to. A pandemic of the proportions of the 1918 pandemic, incidentally, has never materialised again, in spite of the frequency of viral mutations and likelihood of creating new viruses that we have no immunity to and despite dire warnings from the pharmaceutical industry trying to encourage wave upon wave of successive vaccination programs.

12.2 Ebola

Ebola received a lot of publicity in its early days, a devastating disease resulting in external and internal bleeding often leading to death. An illness of which we have no treatment, no knowledge of where the virus normally inhabits, but often associated with health-care facilities and one form can also occur in monkeys, gorillas and chimpanzees. This Ebola-Reston virus was supposed to cause severe illness and death in monkeys imported to research facilities in the United States and Italy from the Philippines; during these outbreaks, several research workers became infected with the virus, but did not become ill.

An illness so devastating, caused by a virus capable of killing anyone in its path, at least that's what the public have been led to believe and yet we have no treatment or vaccine, which raises the question, why hasn't it killed everyone in its path? The source of the virus is unknown;

therefore quarantine would only be possible once the patient had symptoms, why is the disease not spreading from whence it came?

A quote from the Centre for Disease Control (special pathogens branch) sheds a different light:

> *"...researchers do not understand why some people are able to recover and some do not"*

Clearly this is also a case of individual susceptibility, without further research there is much about the illness that remains unknown, however it is interesting to know that it usually spreads within healthcare facilities which are of course immune suppression facilities and in laboratory animals as opposed to other animals in captivity.

12.3 Bird Flu

And so to Bird Flu, reminding me of the saying 'if you want to know the truth, follow the money'. The story is the same, individuals becoming ill and dying, we find evidence of a possible virus in their system and we say that is the cause of their death. The problem is, however, how do we know that the virus is not an effect rather than the cause? Viruses are species specific, meaning that humans do not replicate bird viruses; the illness has only appeared in those in close contact with birds, bird viruses found in humans may have been found as a result of contamination but have no role in pathology.

The living conditions of live stock are important factors in their disease and therefore in the formation of viruses, more important than the theory of catching a disease from the transmission of a virus from another bird, why are we not looking at those conditions when assessing the factors responsible for disease? Why should we be more concerned of the bird flu virus mutating to a human form as compared to any other animal virus on the planet? Birds in captivity are also subject to poisoning which could create viruses; they are also subject to vaccination which does create mutant viruses. Laboratories are in fact altering these bird flu viruses (for example AH5N1) with human influenza viruses, what are the possible implications with regard to vaccinations in humans and live-stock?

Patricia A. Doyle, DVM, PhD., Tropical Agricultural Economics:

"I have been plotting outbreaks for almost two years, using migration maps and studying bird flyways, etc. Well, I noticed something different this season. The winter bird migrations did NOT bring bird flu with the migratory birds. Cases should NOW be breaking out in Africa, Malawi and other countries that host winter migratory birds. Well, the bird flu does not seem to be where it is supposed to be i.e. going by the past migrations…are the re-emerging outbreaks in china, Vietnam, Russia, Romania etc. occurring due to vaccinations?"

We have already mentioned Dr Marc Girard's condemnation of the WHO promotion of a flu vaccine against a predicted pandemic of bird flu:

*"As a result, experts are currently challenging the WHO on the fact that deporting a veterinarian issue to a medical one prevented national agencies from taking appropriate measures concerning animals which, most probably, would have been far more efficient in limiting the spread of epidemics. In addition, it is sufficient to consider the figures of fatal reports following flu vaccination (Scrip n° 3101, p. 6) and to have a minimum of familiarity with the problem of under-reporting, to understand that up till now **irresponsible vaccination against flu has killed far more people than avian (bird) flu."***

And to follow the money, Donald Rumsfeld, USA Secretary of State holds shares in the company 'Gilead' that owns the rights to the so-called anti-viral drug 'Tamiflu', which is being produced under license by the Swiss Pharmaceutical 'Roche', promoted as the drug of choice in any forth coming bird flu epidemic. October 2005, Nelson D.

Schwartz, senior writer of the USA business magazine 'Fortune' reports:

> "Rumsfeld served as Gilead Research's chairman from 1997 until he joined the Bush administration in 2001 and he still holds a Gilead stake valued at between $5 million and $25 million, according to federal financial disclosures filed by Rumsfeld. The forms don't reveal the exact number of shares Rumsfeld owns, but in the past six months fears of a pandemic and the ensuing scramble for Tamiflu have sent Gilead's stock from $35 to $47. That's made the Pentagon chief, already one of the wealthiest members of the Bush cabinet, **at least $1 million richer.**"

Did the pandemic materialise, millions of cases, 1,000's dead? No, it did not, we are of course still waiting for the pandemic, 6 months later however, what did materialise for Donald Rumsfeld?

March 2006, Geoffrey Lean and Jonathan Owen report in the UK newspaper 'The Independent'.

> "Donald Rumsfeld has made a killing out of bird flu. The US Defence Secretary has made more than $5m (£2.9m) in capital gains from selling shares in the biotechnology firm that discovered and developed Tamiflu, the drug being bought in massive amounts by Governments to treat a possible human pandemic of the disease."

So, is the bird flu panic lead by scientific evidence? Apparently not, at least, according to a report in the British Medical Journal.

> "The lack of sustained human-to-human transmission suggests that this AH5N1 avian virus (the bird flu virus) does not currently have the capacity to cause a human pandemic"

> BMJ, Oct 2005, (331: 975 – 976)

12.4 HIV

What about illnesses such as HIV you may say, surely we have a formidable and virulent pathogen indiscriminately attacking and killing those that it happens to infect. From the old infectious disease perspective this may appear to be the case and is certainly promoted as such by the popular press and the proponents of mainstream pharmaceutical approaches to disease management. An analysis of the research is in fact very straight forward in those with a minimum of research background, but a very large subject and too large to do justice to in this book, however I shall quote from the numerous and eminent scientists that are fully aware that the disease phenomena, Acquired Immune Deficiency Syndrome (AIDS), cannot be attributable to a single virus, HIV or any other.

Many scientists within the field of virology and AIDS research have always questioned the role of the newly discovered retrovirus HIV as the causation of the illness AIDS. Indeed after several years of research many are convinced that HIV is not in fact the cause of AIDS and a number of scientists have formed; 'The Group for the Scientific Reappraisal of the HIV-AIDS Hypothesis' and have documented statements and links to research and correspondence stating just that:

Dr. Kary Mullis, Biochemist, 1993 Nobel Prize for Chemistry:

> "If there is evidence that HIV causes AIDS, there should be scientific documents which either singly or collectively demonstrate that fact, at least with a high probability. There is no such document." (Sunday Times - London, 28 Nov. 1993)

Dr. Heinz Ludwig Sänger, Emeritus Professor of Molecular Biology and Virology, Max-Planck-Institutes for Biochemistry, München. Robert Koch Award 1978:

> "Up to today there is actually no single scientifically really convincing evidence for the existence of HIV. Not even once

such a retrovirus has been isolated and purified by the methods of classical virology." (Letter to Süddeutsche Zeitung 2000)

Dr. Serge Lang, Professor of Mathematics, Yale University:

"I do not regard the causal relationship between HIV and any disease as settled. I have seen considerable evidence that highly improper statistics concerning HIV and AIDS have been passed off as science, and that top members of the scientific establishment have carelessly, if not irresponsibly, joined the media in spreading misinformation about the nature of AIDS." (Yale Scientific, Fall 1994)

Dr. Harvey Bialy, Molecular Biologist, former editor of *Bio/Technology* and *Nature Biotechnology*:

"HIV is an ordinary retrovirus. There is nothing about this virus that is unique. Everything that is discovered about HIV has an analogue in other retroviruses that don't cause AIDS. HIV only contains a very small piece of genetic information. There's no way it can do all these elaborate things they say it does." (Spin June 1992)

Dr. Gordon Stewart, Emeritus Professor of Public Health, University of Glasgow:

"AIDS is a behavioural disease. It is multifactorial, brought on by several simultaneous strains on the immune system - drugs, pharmaceutical and recreational, sexually transmitted diseases, multiple viral infections." (Spin June 1992)

Dr. Charles Thomas, former Professor of Biochemistry, Harvard and Johns Hopkins Universities:

"The HIV-causes-AIDS dogma represents the grandest and perhaps the most morally destructive fraud that has ever been

perpetrated on young men and women of the Western world."
(Sunday Times (London) 3 April 1994)

Dr. Joseph Sonnabend, New York Physician, founder of the American Foundation for AIDS Research (AmFAR):

"The marketing of HIV, through press releases and statements, as a killer virus causing AIDS without the need for any other factors, has so distorted research and treatment that it may have caused thousands of people to suffer and die." (Sunday times (London) 17 May 1992)

Dr. Etienne de Harven, Emeritus Professor of Pathology, at the University of Toronto:

"Dominated by the media, by special pressure groups and by the interests of several pharmaceutical companies, the AIDS establishment efforts to control the disease lost contact with open-minded, peer-reviewed medical science since the unproven HIV/AIDS hypothesis received 100% of the research funds while all other hypotheses were ignored." (Reappraising AIDS Nov./Dec. 1998)

Dr. Bernard Forscher, former editor of the U.S. *Proceeding of the National Academy of Sciences*:

"The HIV hypothesis ranks with the 'bad air' theory for malaria and the 'bacterial infection' theory of beriberi and pellagra [caused by nutritional deficiencies]. It is a hoax that became a scam." (Sunday Times (London) 3 April 1994)

Not only are there problems with the HIV causes AIDS hypothesis but astoundingly the evidence for the existence of the newly discovered retrovirus HIV is almost entirely non-existent. Researchers have been working with what they think the retrovirus is doing (i.e. reverse transcription) without ever having isolated and therefore found the virus. In addition when diagnosing someone with having the virus HIV positive, they are in fact detecting antibodies to a protein that they believe is from the virus.

Electron microscopy of the relevant portions of the cells that contain the virus is a minimal requirement of identification; Dr. Etienne de Harven is emeritus Professor of Pathology, University of Toronto. He worked in electron microscopy (EM) primarily on the ultrastructure of retroviruses throughout his professional career of 25 years at the Sloan Kettering Institute in New York and 13 years at the University of Toronto. Regarding HIV research and the lack of electron microscopy studies he has this to say:

> *"It is only in 1997, after fifteen years of intensive HIV research, that elementary EM (electron microscopy) controls were performed, with the disastrous results recently reviewed in Continuum. How many wasted efforts, how many billions of research dollars gone in smoke...**Horrible.**"*

The disastrous results were the first electron micrographs i.e. highly magnified pictures of portions of cell extracts supposed to be containing isolated virus and the discovery that most of the contents was in fact cell debris and smaller particles without the structure of retroviruses. This is what researchers were using as isolated HIV retrovirus.

Most of the scientific community accepts what they are being told by other researchers; most of the non-research scientific community including health professionals accept likewise, and therefore the public, way down the information line, accept what is being perpetuated by the media, hook, line and sinker. When researchers do their own investigating, they are often surprised:

Dr. Heinz Ludwig Sänger, Emeritus Professor of Molecular Biology and Virology and a former director of the Department of Viroid Research at the Max-Planck-Institutes for Biochemy near Munich:

*"During the past 20 years HIV-AIDS research has shown to a line of critical scientists again and again that the existence of HIV has not been proven without doubt, and that both from an aetiological (causal), and an epidemiological view, it can not be responsible for the immunodeficiency AIDS. In view of the general accepted HIV/AIDS hypothesis **this appeared to me so unbelievable that I decided to investigate it myself.** After three years of intensive and, above all, critical studies of the relevant original literature, as an experienced virologist and molecular biologist I came to the following surprising conclusion:*

"... Up to today there is actually no single scientifically really convincing evidence for the existence of HIV. Not even once such a retrovirus has been isolated and purified by the methods of classical virology."

We are of course no different, what choice do we have other than to believe what the scientific community appears to be telling us, albeit through the mechanism of the media. It is therefore important to realise that the HIV/AIDS theory, the theory that you can catch AIDS by catching the HIV retrovirus, is just a theory, to which many scientists do not adhere to and of which the evidence for is entirely lacking. However, the counter story, even though scientifically more dominant, does not get media attention.

Time again throughout history we have witnessed the advent of a disease that is promoted as being caused by a powerful disease agent, something that exists outside of us, that has nothing to do with our own susceptibility, when in fact research shows quite the opposite. In spite of this, research finances are poured into attempting to find the 'one' external microbial cause, so that we can profitably produce the magic bullet and administer cure without the need to take responsibility for a single contributing disease factor. Meanwhile the real factors that determine health and disease are side-lined; - toxicity, nutritional deficiency, suppressed elimination, immune suppression, emotional abuse, emotional suppression and drug use.

AIDS is not in fact a single disease, there are many different symptoms and it is classified differently in different countries, there are now syndromes that look like AIDS that are now called ARC (AIDS Related Complex). The attachment to a belief that disease is caused by an external germ is so strong that it can defy rationality.

> *"The 'rules' employed by HIV/AIDS researchers, that is, detection of a protein, p24, OR an enzyme, reverse transcriptase, do not satisfy any scientific principle proving isolation of a viral particle and indeed **defy common sense"**.*

Written by Dr. Eleni Papadopulos-Eleopulos, Professor of medical physics and Dr. David Causer, Senior physicist, head of medical physics, both at Royal Perth Hospital together with Dr. Valendar Turner, Professor of emergency medicine and Dr. John Papadimitriou, Practicing pathologist and Professor at University both of Western Australia's medical school, in response to the claim that HIV has been found in AIDS patients.

The story of AIDS is an account of disease that once more highlights the ability of those in power to grasp at opportunities to promote their own social agenda and their own financial gain, and for others in research, supported by the same financial institutions, to base investigations that express a limited mindset, whilst satisfying those that are psychologically attached to a simplistic view of disease that has been promoted since the days of Pasteur.

12.5 Swine Flu

12.5.1 Were the dangers of the Swine Flu Vaccine ignored and the risks of the illness exaggerated?

A mass swine flu vaccination programme in the U.S. in 1976 caused far more deaths than the disease it was designed to combat, and the

Health Protection Agency watchdog has asked doctors to look out for cases of Guillain-Barré Syndrome (GBS) when the vaccinations begin.

According to Meryl Nass, M.D., an authority on the anthrax vaccine:

> "A novel feature of the two H1N1 vaccines being developed by companies Novartis and GlaxoSmithKline is the addition of squalene-containing adjuvants to boost immunogenicity and dramatically reduce the amount of viral antigen needed. This translates to much faster production of desired vaccine quantities."

All higher organisms produce the hydrocarbon squalene (oil soluble), including humans. Squalene is a natural and vital part of the synthesis of cholesterol, steroid hormones, and vitamin D in the human body.

The difference between "good" and "bad" squalene is the route by which it enters your body. Injection is an abnormal route of entry which may incite your immune system to attack all the squalene in your body, not just the vaccine adjuvant.
Anti-squalene antibodies have also been linked to Gulf War Syndrome

Symptoms included - arthritis, fibromyalgia, lymphadenopathy, rashes, photosensitive rashes, malar rashes, CFS, headaches, hair loss, non-healing skin lesions, aphthous ulcers, dizziness, weakness, memory loss, seizures, mood changes, neuropsychiatric problems, anti-thyroid effects, anaemia, elevated ESR, lupus, MS, ALS, Raynaud's, chronic diarrhoea, night sweats and low-grade fevers.

How did the authorities assess the safety of the Swine flu vaccine?

Because authorities believe this is and will be a severe pandemic, it is felt that emergency protective measures are needed. It is on the basis of the safety and efficacy record of the existing seasonal flu vaccine programs that the swine flu vaccine program will be fast-tracked through…because there is no time to conduct the usual efficacy and safety tests.

However the safety of the swine flu vaccine cannot be gleaned from old data because the viral elements are new and there will be new adjuvants and new combinations of virus. So if the virus is new enough to cause panic, pandemic and huge death toll, why is it not considered new enough to warrant anything more than traditional rapid testing of the normal flu vaccines.

Swine flu trials

Trialled on healthy 18-50 year olds…however the vaccines will be used on everyone else! Elderly, sick, pregnant and young children.

Can we rely on the safety data from swine flu trials?

Nina Bautz reported in the German newspaper Munich Merkur 21/8/09:

> *Graduate businessman Axel Sch. (40) claims: "The vaccination has made me ill! – the test is irresponsible." He says that within a few hours after the vaccination, on August 10, he had sweat on his forehead. "I felt totally beat. On the third day, my kidneys and head were aching and I got a fever. I then had a coughing fit – and the wash basin was suddenly red – it was blood!"*
>
> *LMU-medical researcher Frank von Sonnenburg, who is in charge of the German country-wide vaccine safety trial, does not consider these accounts credible. He says that such side-effects cannot be related to the vaccine.*
>
> *Axel Sch. however insists that his complaints were a result of the vaccination. "Surely it is no coincidence that they occurred directly after the vaccination."*

Now his trust in research is gone, he is quitting the vaccine trial.

Doctors and Nurses not convinced of the vaccine...

Up to half of family doctors do not want to be vaccinated against swine flu. More than two thirds of those who will turn the jab down believe it has not been tested enough. Most also believe the flu has turned out to be so mild in the vast majority of cases that the vaccine is not needed.

Richard Hoey, editor of Pulse, said: 'The medical profession has yet to be convinced by the Government's whole approach to swine flu, with most family doctors now feeling that the Department of Health overreacted in its policy on blanket use of Tamiflu...initially recommended and later withdrawn from blanket use. Nurses polled also reflect that one third are unwilling to be vaccinated

Will the vaccine be tested?

If authorities can't show effectiveness in 40 years of seasonal flu vaccine how are they going to do it now with swine flu vaccine?

Is the vaccine going to be tested at all? Governments say yes, however they have already bought the vaccines on the basis that the vaccines will pass tests on a certain date.

> *"Therefore: how is it possible to have a pre-specified schedule of approval in a process where the approval may be delayed or even rejected? And how is it possible for governments to spend public funds by paying in advance for products whose introduction on the market may never be granted?*

The answer is clear:

> *Our health authorities have never been seriously thinking of genuinely assessing the new influenza vaccines."*

Dr Marc Girard

Evidence emerging swine flu is a mild illness.

Before the vaccine campaign is underway the evidence emerging from the Southern Hemisphere is that this is an unusually mild illness. Inspite of this evidence pandemic status remains and vaccine promoters urge vaccination to protect against the flu mutating to a more serious form.

However if we do follow this argument we see that it is quite incongruent: Mutation is the tendency of all flu illnesses, therefore what's so special about this one and why is it necessarily more deadly than previous diseases?

If it does mutate it could equally mutate to a less dangerous illness. Additionally if it does mutate significantly the vaccine made from existing swine flu virus would be useless.

Why are people so scared of the swine flu?

Peter Doshi, "Viral Marketing: The Selling of the Flu Vaccine." March. 2006:

> *There is a strategy for selling flu shots. 2004 National Influenza Vaccine Summit, Glen Nowak of CDC explained how certain messages generate buzz and drive demand.*

> *The influenza vaccine is a national industry, with President Bush asking Congress to fund a $7.1 billion "flu preparedness plan."*

> *The recipe, as Nowak revealed, relies on creating "concern, anxiety, and worry" its main ingredient, in other words, is fear. Government officials and health experts are instructed to: "Predict dire outcomes."*

2002 focus group, the CDC determined that death statistics were "eye catching and motivating." Participants in the study believed "20,000 deaths was compelling, frightening" and "should be part of the headline." In 2003, the agency began announcing that the number of Americans killed each year by flu had surged to 36,000, an 80 percent increase that is now widely reported.

Among all flu-prevention messages in the news during the week of 9/21/03, according to Nowak's presentation, "Flu kills 36,000 per year" appeared second most often, just behind "Doctors recommend/urge flu shot."

But the 36,000 figure is actually a measure of "flu-associated" fatalities, almost exclusively among the elderly and infirm, whose deaths from other illnesses the CDC thinks might not have occurred without the flu but not caused by flu. Records show that only 1,400 deaths a year are attributed to flu.

Another way to "motivate behavior," is to describe a flu season as "very severe," "more severe" than previous years, and "deadly" all terms that had been used to frame the 2003-2004 threat. Yet that winter's flu was later ruled "typical" and "medium in terms of overall impact."

The CDC believes anything that encourages more people to get flu shots, even, as suggested in this step, spreading the notion that all of us could be in serious danger, will result in fewer deaths.

But the efficacy of the flu vaccine is itself uncertain. After looking at more than three decades of data, scientists at the National Institutes of Health last year concluded

"We could not correlate increasing vaccination coverage after 1980 with declining mortality rates in any age group." And

because flu shots contain some level of toxic mercury, there is concern that for some the vaccine might do more harm than good.

12.5.2 Why is the effectiveness of Swine Flu vaccine being questioned?

The Swine flu vaccine is going to be manufactured from the technology of existing flu vaccines and therefore requires no new testing, the pandemic status designated by the WHO requires fast-track through production and safety trials.

What is the safety and efficacy record of existing flu vaccines, given the amount of resources used to implement worldwide flu vaccine programs?

Vaccines are given to reduce deaths and incidence of the disease especially in the vulnerable, they often vaccinate the healthy and high contact risk groups to affect herd immunity and protect the vulnerable. However Flu vaccines and Swine Flu vaccine were given to the vulnerable!

People for whom vaccination is recommended in the United States:

Aged 65 or more (and 50-64), children aged 6months – 5years, people with chronic medical conditions, cardiovascular, respiratory conditions (including asthma but excluding hypertension) and compromised ability to eliminate infected excretions. Those treated in hospital in the preceding 12 months for a range of conditions (for example, diabetes or haemoglobinopathy), children aged 6 months to 18 years being treated with aspirin. Women who are pregnant during the influenza "season". Carers and household contacts (including children) of those in the above risk categories and of children aged 0-59 months, healthcare workers.

Evidence of effectiveness:

After an effective flu vaccine campaign, one would expect to see reductions in, cases, admissions to hospital, mortality of elderly people, antibiotic prescriptions and absenteeism.

Dr Tom Jefferson
Head of the Vaccines Field at the Cochrane Collaboration

In choosing illnesses with high antigenic match to vaccine (be kind to the vaccine!) studies in elderly have shown very little effect on **incidence** (no reduction in numbers of cases) but mysteriously reduced **mortality** (somehow reduced deaths due to flu).

It is impossible for a vaccine that does not prevent influenza to prevent its complications; including admission to hospital...A more likely explanation for such a finding is selection bias...

Poor study quality in children; five randomised studies and five non-randomised studies were reviewed, but although data were suggestive of protection, its extent was impossible to measure because of the weak methods used in the primary studies.

In children under 2 years inactivated vaccines had the same field efficacy as placebo. In healthy people under 65, vaccination did not affect hospital stay, time off work, or death from influenza and its complications.

Reviews found no evidence of an effect in patients with asthma or cystic fibrosis, but studies showed inactivated vaccines reduced the incidence of exacerbations after three to four weeks by 39% in those with chronic obstructive pulmonary disease.

One scandalous statistic is that BEFORE the CDC advocated vaccinating children under the age of five, the number of children dying from the flu was very low, and on the decline.

Then, in 2003, just after children aged five and under started getting vaccinated, the number of flu deaths INCREASED significantly. The death toll was enormous compared to the previous year, when the flu vaccine was not administered en masse to that age group.

Influenza deaths under 5

25	19	15	13	90
1999	2000	2001	2002	2003

How can one consider a strategy that yields a higher death toll to be a 'success'?

Were the benefits of the ordinary seasonal flu vaccine grossly exaggerated?

It is stated by vaccine promoters that **flu vaccines reduce deaths in elderly by 50%**. Yet when researchers from the National Institute of Allergy and Infectious Diseases included all deaths from illnesses that flu aggravates, like lung disease or chronic heart failure, they found that **flu accounts for, at most, only 10 percent** of winter deaths among the elderly.

So how could flu vaccine possibly reduce total deaths by half?

Tom Jefferson, a physician based in Rome and the head of the Vaccines Field at the Cochrane Collaboration, a highly respected international network of researchers who appraise medical evidence, says:

> *"For a vaccine to reduce mortality by 50 percent and up to 90 percent in some studies means it has to prevent deaths not just*

*from influenza, but also from falls, fires, heart disease, strokes, and car accidents. **That's not a vaccine, that's a miracle.***"

How do we explain those inflated estimates of vaccine effectiveness?

When Lisa Jackson, a physician and senior investigator with the Group Health Research Center, in Seattle, began wondering aloud to colleagues if maybe something was amiss with the estimate of 50 percent mortality reduction for people who get flu vaccine, the response she got sounded more like doctrine than science.

> *"People told me, 'No good can come of [asking] this,'" she says. "'Potentially a lot of bad could happen' for me professionally by raising any criticism that might dissuade people from getting vaccinated, because of course, 'We know that vaccine works.' This was the prevailing wisdom."*

2004, Jackson and three colleagues set out to determine if there was a "healthy user effect". Are the people getting vaccinated simply healthier than those who don't, people who don't get vaccinated may be bedridden or otherwise too sick to go get a shot.

To test their thesis, Jackson and her colleagues studied eight years of medical data on more than 72,000 people 65 and older. They looked at who got flu shots and who didn't. Then they examined which group's members were more likely to die of any cause when it was not flu season.

Jackson's findings:
Outside of flu season, the baseline risk of death among people who did not get vaccinated was approximately 60 percent higher than among those who did, therefore on average, healthy people chose to get the vaccine, while the "frail elderly" didn't or couldn't.

The 'healthy-user effect' explained the entire benefit that other researchers were attributing to flu vaccine, suggesting that the vaccine itself might not reduce mortality at all.

Lone Simonsen - Professor of global health at George Washington University, Washington, D.C., Internationally recognized expert in influenza and vaccine epidemiology.

> *Jackson's papers "are beautiful," says Lone Simonsen, "They are classic studies in epidemiology, they are so carefully done"*

The results were also so unexpected that many experts simply refused to believe them. Jackson's papers were turned down for publication in the top-ranked medical journals.

One flu expert who reviewed her studies for the Journal of the American Medical Association wrote,

> *"To accept these results would be to say that the earth is flat!"*

When the papers were finally published in 2006, in the less prominent International Journal of Epidemiology, they were largely ignored by doctors and public-health officials.

> *"The answer I got," says Jackson, "was not the right answer."*

Dr Tom Jefferson (Head of the Vaccines Field at the Cochrane Collaboration) summarises the evidence:

1 *Evidence from systematic reviews shows that inactivated vaccines have little or no effect on the effects measured.*

2 *Most studies are of poor methodological quality and the impact of confounders is high.*

3 Little comparative evidence exists on the safety of these vaccines

Dr Marc Girard – expert witness in presenting and assessing vaccine damage cases in France:

All the available relevant flu vaccine studies (randomized controlled trials, cohort and case-control studies) performed from 1966 to 2006, during 40 years shows:

Neither the manufacturers, nor any health agency have produced any convincing evidence of a significant benefit related to vaccines against influenza.

Even more paradoxical since, as everybody knows, available studies are rather skewed towards an overestimation of benefits, because of the publication bias. To say the same in more mathematical way:

If an overestimation of benefits proves to be near zero, at which level may be the real benefits?

12.5.3 Why is big pharma being investigated for its role in the swine flu vaccine scandal?

In this season's pandemic scare, Congress has responded to Bush's call by passing a bill that allows the government to confer blanket immunity from liability on makers of vaccines. As the wages of fear accrue to pharmaceutical companies, Americans are made into a captive market for vaccines of questionable worth

Big Pharma...

Why Did Baxter Patent Hybrid Flu Vaccine a Year Ahead of Outbreak?

Interestingly, despite the fact that health authorities around the world were "shocked" at the emergence of this never-before-seen hybrid flu strain, Baxter had patented a flu vaccine covering these now infamous strains on August 28, 2008.

> Baxter's patent # US2009 0060950 A1 includes "more than one antigen... such as influenza A and influenza B in particular selected from of one or more of the human H1N1, H2N2, H3N2, H5N1, H7N7, H1N2, H9N2, H7N2, H7N3, H10N7 subtypes, of the **pig flu H1N1**, H1N2, H3N1 and H3N2 subtypes, of the dog or horse flu H7N7, H3N8 subtypes, or of the avian H5N1, H7N2, H1N7, H7N3, H13N6, H5N9, H11N6, H3N8, H9N2, H5N2, H4N8, H10N7, H2N2, H8N4, H14N5, H6N5, H12N5 subtypes."

First swine flu case in Mexico didn't emerge until mid-March, 2009, and the mixture of human-avian-swine viruses was considered to be quite an anomaly and not likely to occur through natural mutation.

Three months later, Austrian investigative journalist Jane Burgermeister filed criminal charges against Baxter AG and Avir Green Hills Biotechnology of Austria, for producing and releasing live H5N1 bird flu virus in Feb 2009 in a vaccine alleging it was a deliberate act to cause and profit from a pandemic. Baxter insists it was an accident, most scientists think that such an accident impossible. If it was an accident, why the media quiet, why no regulatory investigation or even criminal proceedings given the potential damage from such negligence?

Swine flu pandemic...what did eventually happen?

The WHO changed the criteria for pandemic status and contracts were awarded to pharmaceutical companies with the patents to provide these vaccines with no damage liability.

Governments spent billions of dollars stock piling vaccines and antivirals for a disease that did in fact turn out to be unusually mild, millions of doses of vaccines were unused and many governments were unable to halt pre-ordered vaccines that were not needed.

But now the European Council is holding an investigation into the role of the WHO and the pharmaceutical industry in promoting undue fear in what was effectively the sales and marketing of patented pharmaceutical products.

Dr Wolfgang Wodard, Chair of the Health Committee in The European Council:

> "We have had a mild flu - and a false pandemic...one of the greatest medical scandals of the century...In January, we will arrange an emergency debate about the influence of the pharmaceutical industry on the WHO, and 47 parliaments all over Europe are going to be informed. Following this, we will initiate an investigation and hearings involving those responsible for the pandemic emergency,"

Paul Flynn Vice chair Council of Europe health comittee came to following conclusion:

> "The world has been subjected to a stunt, for the own greedy interests of the pharmaceutical companies."

> http://www.examiner.com/x-24152-Healthy-Living-Examiner~y2010m1d14-European-Council-investigates-swine-flu-pandemic-hoax

A question that emerges in most peoples minds, often long before this point, is: What would the vaccine expert response be to these general criticisms?

CHAPTER THIRTEEN

13 Top World Health Organisation vaccine expert unable to address the fundamental criticisms of vaccines

So far we have established to some degree that the method of vaccination carries with it potential risks. The procedure itself is designed to stimulate a partial immune response, i.e. blood antibodies; however, as immunologists and health professionals are aware, this partial immune response is **not** the most important aspect of our immune function.

This is illustrated by the fact that, the response to natural disease with the **elimination** of toxins, enhanced membrane function, cellular immune reactions etc, culminating in life-long immunity is not reproduced during the process of vaccination. Furthermore, as a matter of vaccine policy, any associated immune reactions such as fever or inflammation, are indiscriminately and routinely suppressed with pharmaceutical medication.

We therefore see increased membrane permeability, allergies, immune deficiency diseases, illnesses associated with high antibody responses, neurological poisoning and autism, all of which we know vaccines can cause.

Vaccines are supposed to reduce our immune burden and thereby reduce incidence and severity of disease, at a negligible risk to the patient, if all this were true there would of course be ample evidence available to the vaccine experts to back this up. The following correspondence between Dr Clements Director of the Extended Program on Immunisation of the World Health Organisation and myself, illustrates the debate with a professional organisation promoting vaccines.

In writing on behalf of 'The Informed Parent' an organisation established to support parents in their vaccine decisions, I was able to draw the WHO into correspondence so that members of the public could read the pro-vaccine side of the debate. Dr Clements was in fact very cooperative in delineating the pro-vaccine argument using measles vaccine as his example.

His initial letter gave some evidence of safety and efficacy but was of course the standard immunogenicity based evidence i.e. research into the effectiveness of measles vaccine in stimulating antibodies, I of course wanted to know of evidence that proved the vaccine works in reducing actual disease and death rate numbers. Then with regard to safety I wanted to know what studies compared the health of vaccinated and non-vaccinated over an extended period of time, therefore controlled studies given that the safety evidence he cited criticised research into the dangers of vaccines because they were not carefully controlled.

Dr Clements promptly responded by citing various research papers, I was then able to obtain copies of this research and responded to Dr Clements directing certain questions at the WHO pointing out the flaws in their approach using much of the argument set out in this book. This letter was published in "The Informed Parent Newsletter" (Spring 1998), since it is long letter and essentially a shortened summary of some of the arguments delineated in this book, the entire content of that letter which also frames his earlier statements can be found in appendix 1. The following is his response to my letter which is, somewhat revealing:

13.1 The WHO Responds:

WORLD HEALTH ORGANIZATION ORGANISATION MONDIALE DE LA SANTE

Direct Téléphone:	41 (22) 791 4402/2657
Facsimile direct:	41 (22) 791 4193
GPV Internet address:	GPV@who.ch
Internet Address:	clem@who.ch

Mr Trevor Gunn
The Informed Parent
PO Box 870
Harrow
Middlesex
HA3 7UW
Royaume-Uni de Grande-Bretagne

In reply please refer to: EPI 18/180/7
                        CJC/SyS (let02101.doc)
Prière de rappeler la référence:

10 February 1998

Dear Mr Gunn,

Thank you for your long letter dated 16th January. May I complement you on your careful and expansive response to my earlier letter. I very much respect your diligence at looking at the literature and carefully considering the issues.

You ask many questions in the text of your letter which would entail a considerable amount of work on my part to answer. While of great interest to you and me, I am not sure that it really benefits lay audiences. The point is that the Expanded Programme on Immunization continues to believe in the value of child immunization as being of overwhelming value to the human race. Until the unlikely moment we have developed perfect vaccines administered by perfect vaccinators, there will remain problems from time to time. But these problems in no way mitigate against the widespread use of the vaccines. Nonetheless, national policy makers must make wise (and often difficult) decisions on what vaccines to include in the national schedule.

I do not feel that it is the right medium to embark on a scientific point-by-point defense of vaccines. My concession to this is to add that vitamin A administration with immunization is part of EPI's policy.

Yours sincerely,

Dr C.J. Clements
Medical Officer
Expanded Programme on Immunization

CH-1211 GENEVA 27-SWITZERLAND Telegr. UNISANTE-GENEVE Telephone: 41 (22) 791 2111 Fax: 41 (22) 791 0746 CH-1211 GENEVE 27-SUISSE

The content of the reply was as follows:

> *Dear Mr Gunn*
>
> *Thank you for your long letter dated 16th January. May I compliment you on your careful and expansive response to my earlier letter. I very much respect your diligence at looking at the literature and carefully considering the issues.*
>
> *You ask many questions in the text of your letter which would entail a considerable amount of work on my part to answer. While of great interest to you and me, I am not sure that it really benefits lay audiences. The point is that the Expanded Programme on Immunisation continues to believe in the value of child immunisation as being of overwhelming value to the human race. Until the unlikely moment we have developed perfect vaccines administered by perfect vaccinators, there will remain problems from time to time. But these problems in no way mitigate against the widespread use of the vaccines. Nonetheless, national policy makers must make wise (and often difficult) decisions on what vaccines to include in the national schedule.*
>
> *I do not feel that it is the right medium to embark on a scientific point-by point defense of vaccines. My concession to this is to add that vitamin A administration with immunisation is part of EPI's policy.*
>
> *Yours sincerely*
> *Dr C J Clements*
> *Medical Officer, Expanded Programme on Immunisation*

This was certainly a perfect opportunity for Dr Clements and therefore the WHO to state their case for the safety and effectiveness of vaccines; of course many observers interpreted this lack of response as an inability to address the substantive criticism of vaccines. Dr Clements was funded by a multi-million dollar organisation, yet stated that a response would entail a great deal of work, something that I as an individual managed to find unpaid time for, writing on behalf of a non-profit organisation The Informed Parent.

Dr Clements was aware of the controversy surrounding vaccines; he had engaged in a public debate and still chose to avoid responding to my letter, I can only assume that he and consequently the entire might of the WHO are unable to respond to the vaccine critique because the criticisms are true and therefore undeniable.

It is also interesting to note that Dr Clements admits that vitamin A administration with vaccination is part of WHO vaccine policy. Given that studies show:

> *Vitamin A supplementation has been shown to reduce the mortality rate due to measles, in under 2 year olds, by seven times. (BMJ, 1987, 294). Many studies show increase eye problems and deaths in children with vitamin A deficiency.*

How on earth can the effects of the vaccine be separated from the effects of vitamin A supplementation? This is of course indicative of the lack of clarity in the research that is supposed to substantiate the pro-vaccine argument. When vaccines are introduced into developing countries and when they have been historically introduced in developed nations, there have been so many other primary health care measures and socio-economic factors to assess, that no worthwhile conclusions can ever be gained without proper controlled studies.

There are many questions that could equally be asked of all the other vaccines, but the issues are the same and therefore the above correspondence with the WHO can be superimposed on the whole vaccine issue and is indicative of the lack of evidence for safety and effectiveness, when looking at the detailed and broader issues of vaccination.

CHAPTER FOURTEEN

14 How the new understanding of illness provides a more effective and empowering approach to managing your health

14.1 Re- visiting Jenner

If we revisit the period of Edward Jenner, we are told that he experimented with a boy called James Phipps, and gave him the first vaccine, produced from the pustules of cowpox. If the boy James Phipps had resolved this blood poisoning we may have expected the manifestation of some kind of eliminatory rash. This did not occur, so <u>was</u> he left with an unresolved condition or had it been resolved in a manner that may not have been noticed or recorded? From our earlier text we have noted:

> James Phipps was declared immune to smallpox but **died of tuberculosis at the age of 20**. Convinced of the virtue of vaccination Edward Jenner inoculated his 18-month-old son with swinepox, on November 1791 and again in April 1798 with cowpox, he too **died of tuberculosis at the age of 21**.

Having a more holistic understanding of disease, being knowledgeable of the nature of unresolved illness, knowing the consequences of immune failure and deeper chronic disease, Edward Jenner would have known that both James Phipps and his son died of what we know as the deeper 'tubercular disease'. They did not develop the rash of smallpox, but in this instance, due to the nature of the blood poisoning induced by the vaccination procedure, they subsequently developed tuberculosis, their disease was in fact driven deeper, and far from being immunised they were in fact immune compromised.

14.2 Germ theory - old paradigm:

The germ (microbe) is primarily responsible for infectious illness and can be transferred from one person to another. Therefore illness itself can be transferred from one person to another.

New paradigm:

> Germs are the result of disease most live normally within the host, hence the dilemma faced in explaining 'carriers' of disease, clearly most of us have these microbes and have no symptoms of disease. We have reached a point where we are now vaccinating against common microbes that we have a normal tolerance of, for example the meningococcal and Hib vaccines. We also see that illnesses do not follow patterns relating to microbe evolution but directly follow disease conditions of the individual and their susceptibility patterns, therefore they proliferate where there is toxicity, emotional susceptibility, nutritional deficiency, immune suppression, inherited susceptibility and immune failure.

In certain instances microbes can be ingested with decayed food along with their toxins causing symptoms of food poisoning, in addition, normal microbes that inhabit the body can contaminate other parts of the body from injuries, all of these are special cases of microbial contamination (the microbe arriving with the material on which it lives).

The so-called infectious illnesses such as measles, chicken pox, polio, tuberculosis, meningitis, etc are entirely different to these, although the old infectious disease paradigm would like to treat them as though they were the same. Such microbes do not fly around the planet infecting individuals, indiscriminately causing disease.

Although microbes can be cultivated in someone with an illness and transferred from one person to another, there is no illness (even in epidemics) unless there is susceptibility and the illness expressed in the next person will be entirely related to their susceptibility. The range of possible symptoms varies according to the susceptibility of the patient.

14.3 Disease classification - old paradigm:

Different microbes cause their own specific illness and therefore infectious illnesses are classified according to the microbe.

New Paradigm:

> An illness cannot be defined by the microbe alone, the illness is inextricably linked to the patient's susceptibility, for example; many microbes can proliferate in the digestive tract and the symptom response involves vomiting, diarrhoea etc, if the same toxins build in the blood the corresponding blood toxicity would be dealt with by forming a rash. If the same toxins and microbes become more invasive affecting the nervous system, symptoms of septicaemia and neuropathy may result. Consequently the conclusions of Pasteur are ultimately inaccurate in the more important details. Different microbes are associated with very similar illnesses (clinically indistinguishable) and the same microbe is associated with widely different illnesses in different people.

14.4 Dangerous disease - old paradigm:

Some microbes are more dangerous than others and can cause serious illnesses even in healthy individuals.

New paradigm:

> ➤ This is ultimately false; a germ is but a germ and is not a disease; a disease is the culmination of complex symptom reactions within an individual, associated with germs and many other causative factors. The possibility of dangerous germs existing and attacking people causing dangerous diseases irrespective of their susceptibility feeds into our fear and if you look into where this concept is promoted you will nearly always find it is when selling medication both pharmaceutical and natural. Sold on the line that "you never know when it can happen to you, even very healthy people can catch a serious illness". Although I have to agree "you never know when 'it' can happen to you", you do know what kinds of things can happen to you in terms of illness and under what circumstances.

> ➤ You will succumb to illness in a manner that is based entirely on your susceptibility, if you are chronically ill with immune deficiency, then when in crisis you will develop an acute illness and it will be the best response given the conditions you are in. The response will not be the problem in itself; the response could very be the step to increased health. "Yes" the illness could also be the step to worse health, but that would be dependent on the conditions that provoke the response, the conditions are the problem not the response, suppress the response and you could make the situation worse.

> ➤ Getting a serious illness can only happen in seriously ill people or when exposed to severe trauma. In a seriously ill person, toxins and microbes become invasive and this is entirely due to host susceptibility, (the state of health of the patient). Drug companies use the worse case scenario to promote vaccines to everyone, creating the impression that the microbe itself is the element that determines how dangerous a disease is, but it is

your susceptibility that determines how dangerous your condition will be.

14.5 Immunity - old paradigm:

The formation of antibodies to microbes is indicative of an effective immune response, therefore the detection and measurement of antibody levels is a measure of immunity within an individual.

New paradigm:

> The large numbers of antibodies measured by immunologists seem to happen as a last resort in blood toxicity; microbes can be kept in appropriate places in the body without them ever having entered the blood and therefore without the need for detectable levels of antibodies. The general immune system develops from birth and with the increase in capability of immune function the numbers of toxins and microbes capable of entering the blood diminishes. Immunity is a learnt process that develops with age, involving many more systems than just B cells and antibodies. Most people are immune to illnesses associated with the many microbes in and around them and have <u>no</u> associated antibodies.

The concept of presenting microbes (as immune challenges in the form of vaccines) to our blood, assumes that we need to see these microbes in our blood in order to recognise them as foreign and deal with them efficiently in the future. It also assumes that we need to produce antibodies to every possible disease agent that we would like to be immune to, but this is a completely flawed and outdated concept of immunity. Immunologists have demonstrated that the immune system learns from its immediate environment, learns from its own cells and from the natural germs on the body. The immune system is able to recognise non-self and does not need to see something before-hand to know that it is not required.

Vaccines are based on an old theory of immunity that is in fact wrong. The more up to date concepts of immunity also acknowledges that immunity is a whole body response and can only be learnt, the learning is general and does not apply to specific microbes. Therefore we do not need to suffer an illness to be immune and we certainly do not need microbes injected into our blood in order to learn that they are foreign.

There are in fact many new paradigms in health; they acknowledge the interplay of energy and matter, the interconnectedness of all our physical systems, the relationship of mind and body, and the interchange between our own cells and the vast ecosystem of our body's vitally important microbes. If we want to understand immunity we need to understand how the body learns to deal with its environment, in order to understand that, we need to discern how we learn to do anything, from learning to walk, talk, eat, or any number of developmental issues.

The new paradigm also acknowledges that the human body is intelligent and that symptoms are a coordinated attempt to deal with the environment, therefore in finding optimum health we need an optimum environment. Optimum health is the interplay of human activity in the greater ecology of the planet. Complementary and alternative treatments acknowledge why and how we are reacting as well as what we are reacting to, it is a more holistic, respectful, safe and effective method of treatment. This perspective opens many doors to individual well-being and creates possibilities in treatment that are simply closed without it. The difference in outcomes when adopting this new paradigm over a more simplistic treatment of the human being is as different as night and day.

For more details on an integrated understanding of a more up to date immunology and holistic medicine see the follow-up book 'SomaWisdom – The Science of Health and Healing' by Trevor Gunn (www.somawisdom.org)

14.6 Vaccination - a summary

Vaccination is based on an outdated model of disease, assigning the cause of disease to a single microbe. Most microbes that are associated with illness exist in healthy individuals and produce no symptoms of disease; in order to understand the causes of illness it is important to understand the state of individual health that makes one susceptible to illness. In searching for magic bullets pharmaceutical companies would like to believe there are single causes to disease; one specific microbe, one gene or one mal-function, this is virtually never the case, and diseases, as all experience shows, are due to a combination of many factors.

By addressing issues of susceptibility; lifestyle, nutrition, water, toxicity, etc, it is possible to dramatically reduce the susceptibility to, and the severity of, illness: Note the dramatic reduction in severity of measles entirely due to addressing these other factors before vaccines were introduced.

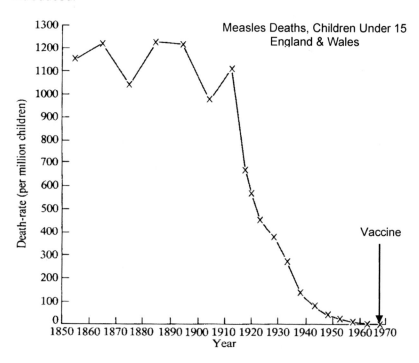

Our understanding of the immune system has developed beyond recognition since the initial conception and development of vaccination; vaccines bypass most of the immune system and push immune responses towards the production of antibodies, this skewed immune response is also indicative of immune dysfunction.

Vaccine safety and effectiveness is estimated without proper controlled studies, without looking at the impact of vaccines on actual disease and longer term health issues. Research shows how vaccines can cause immune disorders, including allergies, autoimmune diseases and even death.

The allergies and immune illnesses associated with vaccines are neither mild nor insignificant; every day 4 people die of asthma in the UK; 1,400 deaths each year across all age groups from asthma alone. Researchers at Children's Hospital Boston found that the number of food-induced allergic reactions treated in their ER more than doubled over six years 2001 – 2006. UK hospital admissions increased seven-fold from 1990 to 2004 as a result of anaphylactic shock a potentially fatal form of allergic reaction.

Vaccine compensation schemes make financial payments to families with children that have died and been damaged by vaccines. Data, disclosed by the Medicines and Healthcare products Regulatory Authority (MHRA) following a request by The Sunday Times under the Freedom of Information Act, shows that from 2003 to 2010, there have been more than 2,100 serious adverse reactions to childhood vaccines and 40 deaths in the UK.

More recently, research conducted by Neil Z Miller and Gary S Goldman published in Human & Experimental Toxicology 2009 (DOI: 10.1177/0960327111407644) shows that, in fact, with developed countries, the more vaccine doses given to their children, the higher the infant death rates. The conclusions of the study were thus:

*It appears that at a certain stage in nations' movement up the socio-economic scale — after the basic necessities for infant survival (proper nutrition, sanitation, clean water, and access to health care) have been met - a counter-intuitive relationship occurs between the number of vaccines given to infants and infant mortality rates: nations with higher (worse) infant mortality rates (i.e. a **higher death rate**) give their infants, on average, **more vaccine doses.***

Neil Z Miller & Gary S Goldman
Human & Experimental Toxicology (2009)

Long term studies looking at disease rates in many individuals choosing not to vaccinate also show health advantages over the vaccinated. Results of researching 6,600 children were reported in the peer reviewed scientific Journal of Allergy & Clinical Immunology in Jan 2006, (Vol.117. No.1) and found that children of Steiner Schools as compared to other children in the same area were significantly less likely to have allergic conditions such as hayfever, eczema and asthma. Here information on environmental exposure, history of infections, diet, animal contact, lifestyle, and use of medication were studied. Importantly it was found that...

*"Reduced use of antibiotics, antipyretics such as calpol, and **reduced MMR vaccine** were found to be associated with a significant reduction in asthma, eczema and hayfever..."*

CHAPTER FIFTEEN

15 Should we be concerned about the accusations from vaccine promoters?

For individuals researching the issues of vaccination I often hear a cry for "wanting the middle ground", torn between what they feel are two extremes of opposing views, there is a desire for reconciling the pro-vaccine and anti-vaccine argument. We inherently know that real life presents issues that require balance, an ability to synthesise opposites and apparent paradox, is it possible that we could vaccinate at some times, in certain individuals for some illnesses…where is the middle-ground?

15.1 Where is the middle-ground?

I would have to agree that all phenomena I have ever come across to date have required the ability to establish equilibrium, not too much and not too little, so where is the middle ground in the vaccine debate?

To know the middle-ground we need first to understand the 'ground', what is the terrain, the terrain of immune development and therefore where are the peripheral extremes so that we can locate the middle? To gain immunity is a whole mind/body learning process and as such, like all learning, involves an encounter with the environment that we have to learn to overcome. This occurs through trial & error and trial & success responses, therefore what are the extremes?

At one end we could present challenges that are very difficult to learn from and therefore very difficult to succeed in overcoming, challenges and traumas that would make us less able to deal with life afterwards.

Toxins, heat, cold, nutritional changes, emotional traumas, in proportions that are too great to overcome, too much too soon, great trauma, high risk, catastrophic failure.

When looking at the issue of immune development, we are considering life from childhood to adulthood and so at the other extreme we could give the individual no stimulus for learning therefore no risk and no possibility of error, no new foods, no space to crawl or walk, no exposure to the outside environment, no separation, always with the mum therefore fostering total dependence, stuck within the present physical and psychological limits, culminating in complete stasis, a breast feeding adult unable to walk or talk. Such scenarios represent the extremes; neither is ideal, both lie at either end of optimum, with their obvious disadvantages.

What therefore is the middle-ground? The slow introduction of stimulus and challenges that enables development, physically, mentally and emotionally; involving trial & error and trial & success responses, with errors that do not precipitate in reduced ability to deal with future challenges but with a large dose of successful outcomes and therefore when there are reactions in error, we allow those reactions to resolve the trauma. Whilst supporting the individual environmentally, physically, nutritionally, mentally, emotionally, to learn to adapt to the environment, with a positive sense of self, health and independence.

Vaccines represent an extreme; trying to mimic the crisis of illness, proposed without an understanding of the terrain, toxic stimulation followed by suppression of any response that could enable learning. This is analogous to teaching a child to cross the road by getting the child run over or rather by trying to mimic the physiological response of the body in a road traffic accident and then suppressing their reactions.

The crisis of a road traffic accident is not a middle path to learning road safety; one does not have to mimic the response of the body in physical trauma in order to teach a child how to cross a road. If a child is hit by a vehicle it is an immediate crisis, it is this we are all trying to avoid.

Learning happens best when there are minimal, albeit consistent, consequences to error.

You can not use vaccines as they are presently designed and tread the middle ground of immune development. Vaccines are by nature extreme, they place poisons beyond most of your immune system and any outward response is then suppressed with pharmaceutical medication. Claiming to be able to use vaccines as a safe method of stimulating the human immune system is a contradiction in terms.

Vaccines are based on wishful thinking they are ultimately dangerous, by using them you are placing the health of yourselves and your children in the hands of the fearful, uninformed and/or commercially motivated. If somebody wishes to vaccinate against a particular illness ask if they understand the meaning of the illness as well as the biological detail; what are the real causes of that illness, what beneficial purpose do the symptoms of that illness serve, what kinds of people are susceptible, have they ever successfully treated people with that illness, what happens if you suppress attempts to resolve the illness, what does the vaccine do and how does it address the causes of the illness? Ask all of the questions that can give you insight and when you are satisfied with the answers then act with courage.

The vaccine debate symbolizes the failure of those that are invested in the bio-mechanical mindset to fully acknowledge the impact of a pharmaceutically driven medical system; one that values money over and above what is best for the patient and on the basis of what is clearly an outdated model of the human being. For some it is a genuine inability to see outside of the paradigm, for others it is a conscious decision to look the other way and yet for others a determined manipulation of the facts, which is borne out of the desire to be right, to avoid change, and to maintain power.

> *"You can't reason someone out of a position they didn't reason themselves into."*
>
> *Author Unknown*

Apathy, fear and greed all play their part, aspects of the human condition fully present in all walks of life. The status quo of any established structure will have some advantages and some distinct disadvantages, the problems with vaccines point to flaws within the system, flaws that unfortunately reach all the way down to the foundations. These limitations are becoming more and more apparent even for those within the system. Jon Rappoport investigative journalist can be found at www.nomorefakenews.com, his interview with a retired vaccine researcher is especially poignant:

> …*Q: In your years working in the vaccine establishment, how many doctors did you encounter who admitted that vaccines were a problem?*
>
> *A: None. There were a few, researchers working within drug companies, who privately questioned what they were doing. But they would never go public, even within their companies.*
>
> *Q: What was the turning point for you?*
>
> *A: I had a friend whose child died after a DPT shot.*
>
> *Q: Did you investigate?*
>
> *A: Yes, informally. I found that this child was completely healthy before the vaccination. There was no reason for his death, except the vaccine. That started my doubts. Of course, I wanted to believe that the child had got a bad shot from a bad lot. But as I looked into this further, I found that was not the case in this instance. I was being drawn into a spiral of doubt that increased over time. I continued to investigate. I found that, contrary to what I thought, vaccines are not tested in a scientific way.*
>
> *Q: What do you mean?*
>
> *A: For example, no proper long-term studies are done on any vaccines using a control group. Part of what I mean is, no correct and deep follow-up is done, taking into account the fact that vaccines can induce, over time, various symptoms and serious problems which fall outside the range of the disease for which the person was vaccinated. Again, the assumption is made that vaccines do not cause problems. So why should*

anyone check? On top of that, a vaccine reaction is defined so that all bad reactions are said to occur very soon after the shot is given. But that does not make sense.

Q: Why doesn't it make sense?

A: Because the vaccine obviously acts in the body for a long period of time after it is given. A reaction can be gradual. Deterioration can be gradual. Neurological problems can develop over time. They do in various conditions, even according to a conventional analysis. So why couldn't that be the case with vaccines? If chemical poisoning can occur gradually, why couldn't that be the case with a vaccine which contains mercury?

...Q: What is one thing you want the public to understand?

A: That the burden of proof in establishing the safety and efficacy of vaccines is on the people who manufacture and license them for public use. Just that, the burden of proof is _not_ on you or me. And for proof you need well-designed, long-term studies. You need extensive follow-up. You need to interview mothers and pay attention to what mothers say about their babies and what happens to them after vaccination. You need all these things - the things that are not there....

...Q: Is there any way to compare the relative frequency of these different outcomes?

A: No. Because the follow-up is poor, we can only guess. If you ask, out of a population of a hundred thousand children who get a measles vaccine, how many get the measles and how many develop other problems from the vaccine, there is no reliable answer. That is what I'm saying. Vaccines are superstitions. And with superstitions, you don't get facts you can use. You only get stories, most of which are designed to enforce the superstition. **But, from many vaccine campaigns we can piece together a narrative that does reveal some very disturbing things.** People have been harmed. The harm is real, and it can be deep and it can mean death. The harm is not limited to a few cases as we have been led to believe. In the US, there are groups of mothers who are testifying about autism and childhood vaccines. They are coming forward and standing up at meetings. They are essentially trying to fill in the gap that has been created by the researchers and doctors who turn their backs on the whole thing.

Q: How long did you work with vaccines?

A: A long time, longer than ten years.

Q: Looking back now, can you recall any good reason to say that vaccines are successful?

A: No, I can't. If I had a child now, the last thing I would allow is vaccination. I would move out of the state if I had to. I would change the family name. I would disappear, with my family. I'm not saying it would come to that. There are ways to sidestep the system with grace, if you know how to act. There are exemptions you can declare, in every State, based on religious and/or philosophic views. But if push came to shove, I would go on the move.

Q: And yet there are children everywhere who do get vaccines and appear to be healthy.

A: The operative word is "appear". What about all the children who can't focus on their studies? What about the children who have tantrums from time to time? What about the children who are not quite in possession of all their mental faculties? I know there are many causes for these things, but vaccines are **one** cause. I would not take the chance. I see no reason to take the chance. And frankly, I see no reason to allow the government to have the last word. Government medicine is, from my experience, often a contradiction in terms. You get one or the other, but not both.

Q: So we come to the level playing field.

A: Yes. Allow those who want the vaccines to take them. Allow the dissidents to decline to take them. But, as I said earlier, there is no level playing field if the field is strewn with lies. And when babies are involved, you have parents making all the decisions. Those parents need a heavy dose of truth. What *about the child I spoke of who died from the DPT shot? What information did his parents act on? I can tell you it was heavily weighted. It was not real information.*

Q: Medical PR people, in concert with the press, scare the hell out of parents with dire scenarios about what will happen if their kids don't get shots.

A: They make it seem a crime to refuse the vaccine. They equate it with bad parenting. You fight that with better information. It is always a challenge to buck the authorities. And only you can decide whether to do it. It is every person's responsibility to make up his or her mind.

The medical cartel likes that bet. It is betting that the fear will win.

The very existence of the vaccine debate is a direct consequence of the suppression of evidence and lack of investment in suitable trials. Ultimately this is the responsibility of governments, health authorities and vaccine producers.

> *"That the burden of proof in establishing the safety and efficacy of vaccines is on the people who manufacture and license them for public use. Just that, the burden of proof is **not on you or me**."*

There are in fact many elements that people take into their bodies and activities that people carry out that will be of benefit to their health, many of which will not have been placebo-control trialed, this would in fact be next to impossible. How do you placebo control trial some of the important things in health and well-being; laughter, music and nature, as well as food quality, sleep, fulfilling work, friends and love, but these things fall under the remit of our life's learning and we are free to make these choices. But in a desperate attempt to side-step the very important issue of vaccine trials, promoters often ask those that question the role of vaccines to provide placebo-controlled evidence for their own position.

This is an argumentative slight of hand, a vaccine is a potentially lethal cocktail of chemicals that do kill individuals, and public funds are used to mass medicate people with these drugs worldwide. The precautionary principle, which is the patently logical principle, requires that they need to prove that vaccines are safe and effective. The onus is not on others to prove this one way or the other; neither does anyone else have to come up with an alternative that is placebo control trialed in order that we question the role of vaccines in health policy. The vaccine debate is not a vaccine versus alternative medicine competition, a specific alternative would of course be nice but not a pre-requisite to the use or not of vaccines, because quite simply it is very possible and of course very likely that vaccines do more harm than good, as afore mentioned studies illustrate, it may be enough to stop vaccinating to increase health and well-being.

Meanwhile, in lieu of properly conducted vaccine trials, enough information is clearly accessible for those that decide to look, and a positive path of self-empowerment is available for those that choose to journey and learn.

> "Everything you're against can be restated in a way that puts you in support of something. Instead of being against war, be for peace. Instead of being against poverty, be for prosperity. Instead of joining a war on drugs, be for purity in our youth.
>
> ...Conflict is a violation of harmony. If you participate in it, you're part of the problem, not the solution."
>
> Wayne Dyer

The way to avoid illness is to understand the ways of health and then illness ceases to be something we run away from or run towards.

CHAPTER SIXTEEN

16 Is this debate simply about the forces of good versus evil?

"As well consult a butcher on the value of vegetarianism as a doctor on the worth of vaccination."

George Bernard Shaw

16.1 Follow the money

The first issue is of course that the employers and employees in the vaccine business, i.e. the pharmaceutical industry, have a duty to make money, for themselves and their shareholders, which has often been shown to take precedence over drug safety and effectiveness:

For example the pharmaceutical company Pfizer was found guilty of illegally promoting the drug bextra for acute pain from surgery, a use that the FDA had already rejected as being unsafe. Pfizer effectively ignored the FDA ruling and with billions of dollars of profits to be made, their marketing and sales teams targeted anesthesiologists, foot surgeons, orthopedic surgeons and oral surgeons.

Pfizer paid out approximately $2billion in fines and compensation after being found guilty but they were deemed too big to be subjected to the appropriate criminal proceedings. Because any company convicted of a major health care fraud is automatically excluded from Medicare and Medicaid. Convicting Pfizer on Bextra would prevent the company from billing federal health programs for any of its products. Drew Griffin and Andy Segal reported on CNN Saturday, Apr 3, 2010

*Prosecutors said that excluding Pfizer would most likely lead to Pfizer's collapse, with collateral consequences: disrupting the flow of Pfizer products to Medicare and Medicaid recipients, causing the loss of jobs including those of Pfizer employees who were not involved in the fraud, and **causing significant losses for Pfizer shareholders**.*

*But after years of overseeing similar cases against other major drug companies, Mike Loucks, the federal prosecutor who oversaw the investigation, **isn't sure $2 billion in penalties is a deterrent** when the profits from illegal promotion can be so large.*

*"I worry that the money is so great," he said, that dealing with the Department of Justice may be **"just the cost of doing business."***

It is very clear that the pharmaceutical giants have a duty to make money, doing this both legitimately and illegally, they have become so large that their activities are very difficult to regulate even when they are convicted of criminal behaviour. Their agenda will of course determine the messages they put out to health professionals and the general public and they have ways of directly influencing both.

16.2 Drug companies now influence local, national and international health agencies?

In their drive for profit and market domination pharmaceutical companies have effectively hijacked the aims and objectives of doctors and health authorities. Many physicians and in fact government health authorities are, sadly, pawns in a billion dollar commercial industry:

Dr Marc Girard was commissioned as an expert medical witness by the French Judge residing over compensation claims for the families of those that died soon after receiving the Hepatitis B vaccine in France. This was the aftermath of a national Hepatitis B vaccine campaign conducted in September 1994 upon the recommendations of the World Health Organisation. The WHO is supposedly a trusted and apparently autonomous organisation with the reputation of being impervious to commercial interests, its sole function is to research and implement policies designed to increase the health and reduce the disease rates of the world's populations.

Dr Marc Girard spent 1000's of hours on the subject with access to dozens of confidential documents, unfortunately what he found, in simple terms, was that the WHO had grossly overplayed the dangers of the actual disease hepatitis B and profoundly underplayed the dangers of the Hepatitis B vaccine. Dr Marc Girard had unearthed an efficient web of coercion exerted by the commercial manufacturers of the vaccine under the auspices of the WHO, in his letter to the Director General of the WHO he states.

> "It is blatant that in the promotion of the hepatitis B vaccination, the WHO has never been more than a screen for an undue commercial promotion, in particular via the Viral Hepatitis Prevention Board (VHPB), created, sponsored and infiltrated by the manufacturers (Scrip n° 2288, p. 22). In Sept 1998, while the dreadful hazards of the campaign had been given media coverage in France, the VHPB met a panel of "experts", the reassuring conclusions of which were extensively announced as reflecting the WHO's position: yet some of the participants in this panel had no more "expertise" than that of being employees of the manufacturers, and the vested interests of the rest did not receive any attention."

Dr Marc Girard found further direct evidence of the ability of vaccine promoters to directly influence the WHO guidelines for their own profit in an interview published in a French Scientific Journal (Sciences et Avenir, Jan 1997: 27).

> "Beecham's business manager claimed with outrageous cynicism "We started increasing the awareness of the

> *European Experts of the World Health Organization (WHO) about Hepatitis B in 1988. From then to 1991, we financed epidemiological studies on the subject to create a scientific consensus about hepatitis being a major public health problem. We were successful because in 1991, WHO published new recommendations about hepatitis B vaccination".*

Dr Girard therefore concludes:

> *It is sad news for people everywhere in the world that the WHO's experts needs manufacturers' salesmen to become aware of significant health problems. As a complementary check, you may be interested to learn that I was personally informed by the journalist responsible for this interview that the manufacturer did its best to prevent the publication of this stunning confession."*

Surprisingly he discovered a similar deception in India reported in The Lancet 2004; 363: 659 by Dr Puliyel:

> *"In Feb 2004, I read a correspondence by an Indian colleague, Dr J. Puliyel (Lancet 2004; 363: 659), on the fallacies of the data spread by the WHO about the epidemiology of hepatitis B in his country.*
>
> *Although not well informed about the health situation in India, I was struck by the fact that the mechanisms of the deception as described by Dr Puliyel (gross exaggerations, lack of references, inappropriate extrapolations), were exactly comparable to those I observed in my own country - and of course with the same results: a plea of "experts" to include hepatitis B vaccination in the national vaccination program, in spite of its cost and, I may add, of its unprecedented toxicity."*

Further observations revealed that these were not isolated incidences, in his research Dr Girard was then able to see a parallel with another disease making the headlines at that time, 'avian flu' otherwise known as 'bird flu'.

> It is quite easy to reconstruct that, under the lame pretext of increasing the manufacturing potential, the manufacturers managed to induce the WHO's experts to recommend flu vaccination, whereas it is plain that this immunization would have no protecting effect against avian flu.

> In both situations, the trick was the same: to create a false alarm (about the inefficiency of targeted vaccination in the case of hepatitis B, about the necessity of increasing the manufacturing process in the case of avian flu), and to induce the WHO to plea for measures based upon misleading recommendations towards lay people (that everybody was at risk of hepatitis B in the former case and that flu vaccination could be useful in the case of avian flu)."

There are of course consequences to 'WHO' policy, their advice influences governments, and these governments, on the basis of this advice, set their own National Health Policies. Doctors and health personnel act on the guidance of that policy and they do so in the belief that the benefit of these vaccines outweighs their risk, they do not carry out further research and their advice to you the public is effectively the filtered down sales promotion from vaccine producers.

The aim of the vaccine producers is clearly to make more and more money; unfortunately this appears to take precedence over and above the recommendation of safe and effective health policy. Dr Marc Girard is not alone in his condemnation of the WHO.

> "As a result, experts are currently challenging the WHO on the fact that deporting a veterinarian issue to a medical one prevented national agencies from taking appropriate measures concerning animals which, most probably, would have been far more efficient in limiting the spread of epidemics. In addition, it

*is sufficient to consider the figures of fatal reports following flu vaccination (Scrip n° 3101, p. 6) and to have a minimum of familiarity with the problem of under-reporting, to understand that up till now **irresponsible vaccination against flu has killed far more people than avian flu.**"*

Dr Marc Girard and Dr Puliyel are calling for an independent enquiry into the nature of WHO vaccine recommendations, in a letter to the Director General of the WHO, Dr Girard concludes:

"...the credibility of your organisation is highly dependent on an inquiry which differentiates between world health interests and those of WHO's experts."

History has of course repeated itself, as I am now, as I return to the content of my opening paragraphs. The more recent handling of the swine flu pandemic of 2009 has all the hallmarks of the previous vaccination campaigns, with overt fear mongering and drive for universal vaccine uptake.

By the spring of 2010 with the predictions of the pandemic dismally wrong the Council of Europe launched an investigation into whether the World Health Organization (WHO) "faked" the swine flu pandemic to boost profits for vaccine manufacturers. The inquiry, held in Strasbourg, France, vindicates a worldwide movement of insiders, experts and elected officials who accuse the United Nations organization of misleading the world into buying millions of unnecessary vaccines.

The opinion given by Dr. Wolfgang Wodarg, an epidemiologist who formerly led the health committee for the Council of Europe is that the WHO changed their criteria for defining pandemic levels to boost vaccine sales.

"There is no other explanation for what happened. Which reasons could lead to those [WHO] decisions? I don't find any other explanation. It's not for health. And who profits? Why else would you change the definition?"

Paul Flynn (Vice Chairman - Council of Europe Health Committee)

"...The world has been subjected to a stunt for their own greedy interests of the pharmaceutical companies"

Clearly pharmaceutical companies have repeatedly used the same tactics to manipulate health professionals and pubic opinion, despite repeated calls for investigations and changes. It would seem logical that they would do this again, surely we must ask ourselves how can this ongoing situation be rectified and in the interim, do we want ourselves and our children to be subjected to any more pharmaceutical stunts?

16.3 Outmoded world view

The fundamental problem however lays in an outmoded world view and the attachment to that belief system with an inability to put that belief system to the ultimate test.

From the outset, the design of vaccine studies themselves are limited by the belief that vaccines work, researchers then try to look back at what effects vaccines have on individuals without the comparison of a control group, a non-vaccinated group, which is of course very difficult to do.

Individual researchers are aware of the restrictions of these retrospective vaccine studies and do seem to do their level best to circumvent these limitations, but there is only so much they can achieve given their specific remit. They know that more trustworthy answers could be attained with properly controlled trials, comparing vaccinated and non-vaccinated.

They are of course blinded by their own faith in vaccines, a belief that the advantages of vaccines outweigh the disadvantages without ever having conducted the definitive trials to assess that conviction.

> *I think the bottom line is that while the zero group is different, and I think all of us would agree with that, the issue is that it is impossible, unethical to leave kids unimmunized, so you will never, ever resolve that issue. So then we have to refer back from that.*
>
> Dr Chen
> Chief of Vaccine Safety & Development
> National Immunization Program, CDC

Researchers are also employed by health agencies that promote vaccination, in the belief that the benefits of vaccines outweigh the disadvantages and consequently have a duty to vaccinate. Therefore when looking at single pieces of evidence that could undermine public confidence in vaccines, they are afraid of the implications and will defend vaccines if on balance they fear it could cause the rejection of a vaccine. Dr Clements head of the WHO vaccine program had this to say when looking at the evidence that vaccines were causing brain and nervous system problems:

> *"My mandate as I sit here in this group is to make sure at the end of the day that 100,000,000 are immunized with DTP, Hepatitis B and if possible Hib, this year, next year and for many years to come..."*
>
> Dr Clements, WHO

The belief in the value of vaccines allows vaccine promoters to reject the individual pieces of research demonstrating vaccine dangers and ineffectiveness, each separate piece of research appears insignificant on its own and so time and again each element is rejected and labeled insignificant compared to the overall value of vaccination as supported by the consensus belief. However it is in fact the overall picture that is being lost by the fragmented view of orthodoxy.

The outmoded world view

These perceptual shortcomings are not unique to medicine; our current and dominant world view is responsible for many of the advantages of 21st century life but also responsible for many of its failings. The dominant belief system is by and large mechanical, linear and simplistic; it underpins agriculture, food production, manufacturing, energy production, politics and many more facets of modern living. But it is also responsible for depleting resources without a strategy for sustainability; killing organisms without a concern for the impact on the larger ecosystem; dividing nations, life forms and the environment into them and us, thereby combating, poisoning and exploiting our world without considering the wider implications.

The Pachamama Alliance is a U.S. based not-for-profit organization looking at the destruction of the rainforests and recognise that it is driven by a complex web of social and economic forces, many of these forces are a logical result of modern society's worldview, a view that, although rich in technological insight, is often ignorant of the value of nature's apparently free and limitless services. They have created a symposium called "Awakening the Dreamer" that is also used by the organisation 'Be the Change' which helps individuals, organisations and cultures to make the changes critical to rebalancing some of the failings in many areas of modern life.

The description of the problems faced by many organisations also accurately reflect the problems with the dominant orthodox medical paradigm, the call for change and assessment of the problem moves away from conspiracy, malice and blame, towards a process of evolving from a fragmented and limited perception to a wider perspective whilst also incorporating technological advancement.

Awakening the Dreamer
It is as if we are living inside of a dream, sleepwalking toward oblivion, while self-serving, shortsighted interests encourage

our slumber with managed news, celebrity culture and other weapons of mass distraction.

It has become clear that our political and commercial institutions are unable to effectively address this crisis, primarily because they don't realize that they are looking at an interconnected world through a fragmented lens. The villain here is not Big Business, the corporate media, the military-industrial complex, or even those who for personal profit seek to clear-cut our forests, overfish our oceans, pollute our atmosphere or drain our aquifers. The villain is an outmoded worldview - a way of seeing the world in which such unthinkable acts appear reasonable, sensible, and even intelligent.

Likewise a medical paradigm where vaccines containing, mercury, aluminium, preservatives, foreign DNA, toxins and antigens, are injected into babies, with subsequent drug suppression of any symptom reactions, appears reasonable, sensible and even intelligent.

The awaken the dreamer symposium has developed out of a need to integrate the details of our technological way of life into the bigger picture, recognising that all of creation is interconnected and each of us is an integral element in this miraculous and fragile weave of life.

The parallels with the shortcomings of our orthodox medical world are striking, where there is a similar need to integrate the knowledge of molecules, cells and symptoms of the body with our own internal microbial ecosystems. Together with the importance of understanding the purpose of symptoms as they relate to the intelligence of the body in keeping us alive and our relationship with the wider environment.

CHAPTER SEVENTEEN

17 What next?

17.1 Does this mean I have to discard orthodox medicine?

It is reasonable to deduce that it is not feasible to get the best health-care by using one approach in all circumstances, however, people often feel pressured to use orthodox medicine and vaccines because they don't want to be abandoned by the medical system.

But it is possible to use the best of all worlds for the health of you and your family, choosing the aspects that you require from each approach; orthodox medical diagnosis, biochemical assessments, surgery, trauma interventions and some medicines are useful approaches when used appropriately. It is also possible to address diet, toxicity and lifestyle issues that reduce susceptibility to illness and use other alternative heath interventions that have been proven to work through your own experience or from others that you trust.

17.2 You are going to need an additional and different type of health care practitioner

In providing optimum health care it is likely that you will need the help of holistic health practitioners as well as the resources of orthodox practitioners; there are many safe and effective strategies to increase health and reduce susceptibility to illnesses provided by many different kinds of practitioners, an effective mix is a more effective option than the limited resources and perspectives delivered solely by orthodox medicine.

The follow-up book 'SomaWisdom – The Science of Health and Healing' (www.somawisdom.org) looks at how we can understand what the body is doing in disease from a more up to date biology and how that integrates with the principles of holistic medicine. This enables individuals to approach their own health care with more effective and safer strategies and understand how to enroll the help of appropriate therapists in dealing with their health challenges.

17.3 The importance of ongoing support to keep on track

It is also vital to realise that there are emotional and cultural reasons for adopting certain attitudes, beliefs and strategies for dealing with illness, for many individuals it is just as significant to understand these issues as well as the basic medical information.

In making improvements in health and adopting new, more effective, strategies it may therefore be necessary to understand which methods are really working for you and which are merely outdated habits that are now inappropriate.

The public and health professionals alike are also subjected to a pervasive and a continual bombardment of messages both overt and more subtle, through the established media and conventional medical channels. Commercial motives may be behind many of these messages and they often prey on the fear of the public. It is important to maintain a perspective of these statements with a balance of the alternatives; therefore ongoing support and up to date information is very often an essential component of what is required to maintain a healthy lifestyle.

Hopefully the content of this book, for many, will be just the start of a process into a deeper and more empowering journey, resolving issues of health and disease and opening new avenues to optimal well-being.

Appendix 1

RESPONSE TO W.H.O. EVIDENCE FOR VACCINE SAFETY AND
EFFECTIVENESS

*Trevor Gunn, BSc Hons, RSHom, corresponding on behalf of The
Informed Parent has forwarded a series of questions to Dr. C. J.
Clements, EPI, Global Programme for Vaccines and Immunisation, of
the World Health Organisation (WHO). Replies have thus created an
opportunity for dialogue on the issue of immunisation safety and
effectiveness. A response to Dr Clements reply has been recently sent
and the following, summarises the points raised ie: the inadequacies in
vaccine testing and the inadequacies in the rationale behind mass
immunisation. We shall of course be happy to print follow-up responses
from the WHO when available. (Informed Parent)*

Many measles vaccine efficacy studies relate to their ability to stimulate an
antibody response, (sero-conversion or sero-response). An antibody response
does not necessarily equate to immunity, the WHO was asked for evidence
showing how sero-response relates to protection in a real disease situation. Dr
Clements thought we were implying that "whatever seroconversion level is
measured, there will be no protection".

However that was not the case, the point being made was that the level of
antibody needed for effective immunity is <u>different</u> in each individual and as
Dr. Clements agreed, immunity can be demonstrated in individuals with a <u>low
or no detectable levels of</u> antibody.

Similarly in other individuals with higher levels of antibody there may be no
immunity. We therefore need to stay clear on the issue: How do we know if
the vaccine is effective for a particular individual when we do not know what
level of antibody production equals immunity?

Dr. Clements agreed, "...there is not a precise relationship between
seroresponse and protection...". This places a greater reliance on obtaining
efficacy results of immunisation from population studies. In the UK the

government Health Authority quotes figures of the measles vaccine as being 90% effective.

Inevitably this leads us to ask the question; 90% effective in doing what? Reducing incidence by 90%? Reducing severity by 90%? Reducing death rate by 90%? Creating antibodies in 90%?

It does in fact mean that, 90% of the recipients of the vaccine, produce a certain level of antibodies to the viral agents in the vaccine, 10% have produced no or undetectable levels of antibody. This information has NOT been derived from population studies and as we have already acknowledged, this does NOT indicate what percentage of those people are actually immune, (or, for that matter, how long that apparent immunity lasts).

So, to state that the vaccine is 90% effective is somewhat misleading and at any rate inaccurate with regard to a statement of immunity in a real disease situation. Therefore the question of vaccine effectiveness can only be answered by population studies that, as stated by Dr. Clements, "do not concern themselves with the response of the individual, rather the protection afforded against the disease to the population immunised".

Dr Clements has therefore quoted references to such studies. Unfortunately they are all studies in developing countries, and as noted in the same studies, the results cannot be directly extrapolated to developed countries. The fear of many individuals in the UK faced with the decision to immunise, is that the risks of vaccination may be greater than that of diseases such as measles, in countries of the developed world. We should like to know of such studies in the so-called developed world and why so few, if any, have been carried out.

We shall nevertheless look at five of the seven studies referenced, as it can sometimes be possible to make worthwhile comparisons with other countries. (One study omitted, P. Canrelle et al, Eds. Paris, as this has proved difficult to obtain in the UK, but again looks at survival rates in a developing country, Senegal, Africa. Also the reference Bolotovski et al, only looks at the difference in antibody responses comparing different types and concentrations of vaccine, and does not compare vaccinated with non-vaccinated).

Reference: P.Aaby et al, Pediat Infec DisJ 8:197-200,1989

This paper looks at the impact of measles vaccination on childhood death rate, (childhood mortality), in Bandim, Guinea-Bissau, Africa. The study acknowledges that if it can be demonstrated that the vaccine is safer than natural measles and is reasonably effective in reducing the incidence of measles, there are still two possible impacts that measles vaccine could have on childhood mortality. On the one hand the weakest children are likely to die from any number of infections, if measles vaccination could prevent measles and therefore measles related deaths, it may still create no overall reduction in mortality as children would be as likely to die from another infection. On the other hand if measles itself causes weakness and malnutrition, effective measles vaccination could lead to a reduction in deaths.

Studies exist that appear to support both theories. Supporters of vaccine programmes adhere to the view that measles vaccination does effectively reduce childhood mortality. However this paper does acknowledge the fact that the vaccinated and unvaccinated groups are NOT strictly comparable in any of the studies supporting this view.

By comparing groups of children with apparently different vaccination status, this study suggests that measles vaccination reduces mortality by 30%.

However, their comparisons in this study would lead one to have serious misgivings about their conclusions. The group used as a "non-vaccinated" group were in fact vaccinated between certain dates. They were found to have undetectable levels of antibody and therefore it was assumed that the vaccine did not work, hence this was used as a 'control' non-vaccinated group.

Most of a second group of 123 individuals, vaccinated at another time were found to have responded and were therefore used as the vaccinated group. However 15 of this vaccinated group did not seroconvert and they were excluded from the results! Three of these children died!

In trying to assess the effectiveness of a vaccine in populations exposed to real disease situations, it will obviously be very misleading to exclude those that do not apparently seroconvert. These may constitute the very percentage of those that suffer adversely in the real disease situation. Therefore results excluding these individuals may obviously favour the effectiveness of the vaccine.

Reference: Clemens et al, American J Epidem Vol 128, No. 6, 1330-39
This study looked at the impact of measles vaccination on childhood mortality in rural Bangladesh. Again the study acknowledges the fact that groups looked at were not strictly comparable for many reasons stated in the paper. In addition one factor overlooked was the effect of selecting individuals for vaccination on the basis of having apparently lacked a history of measles. This may select out those that have had measles at a young age and using the same rationale expressed in the study, these may well be the weaker section of the community most likely to die of measles or go on to die from underlying comorbid illnesses aggravated by contracting measles at an early age.

The paper goes on to say that their results cannot necessarily be extrapolated to programs in other countries, where measles vaccine may be given according to different age criteria or where a different relation may exist between measles and the subsequent risk of death.

Reference: Koenig et al, Bulletin of WHO 68 (4): 441-447 (1990)
This was an extension of the above previously quoted study conducted at the same centre in rural Bangladesh. Again concentrates on survival, defining a period of three years as a long term study.

Reports from studying two periods were given, one found a reduction of mortality of 46%, the other 36%. One of the reasons given for this difference was that, an area from which non-vaccines were drawn experienced higher childhood mortality than the vaccinated area as a result of a localised outbreak of dysentery. Consequently the vaccine appeared to be more effective than might otherwise have been.

This highlights the difficulty in using separate areas with different localised disease conditions for comparing the effects of vaccination. Again the report states that caution must be exercised in extrapolating the results of the present study to settings other than Bangladesh.

Reference: E. Holt et al, Paediatrics Vol.85, No 2, p188-194, Feb 1990
This was a study of the effect of measles vaccination on childhood mortality in a pen-urban slum in Tahiti. This showed much higher rates of reduction in mortality. It was not so clear as to why this was the case. It was suggested that the earlier age of vaccination compared to other studies could have been responsible. This is , 9 months (studied over a period of 30 months), as compared to 10 months (studied over a period of 40 months). It does seem hard to imagine why this difference of one month should make such a large difference in survival.

There was no mention in the paper that this may also relate to the shorter period studied. It has been reported that "gains in survival of a vaccinated group tend to diminish over time to approach a survival rate of unvaccinated individuals". (The lancet April 4, 1981 765). The weakest children most at risk go on to die from other infections, (as discussed in the first paper above, P.Aaby et al Ped Inf Dis).

This study does show, however, that socio-economic factors make a huge difference with regard to childhood survival. Improvements in living standards having almost as much an effect on reducing mortality as that predicted using vaccination.

Given the interest of the WHO in responding to questions, and their desire to show convincing evidence, one would assume that these studies were some of the better ones. Yet as we can see, they are sadly inadequate.

The last paper goes on to state, (as have others), that "the definitive test of the papers hypothesis would require a prospective randomised placebo-controlled trial that we believe would be unethical". We shall therefore look at the issue of a placebo-controlled trial and the question of ethics.

Double-blind placebo-controlled trial.
This involves a comparison of the results from a placebo group, (a group of individuals that do not take the active medication), with an equivalent group that have had the active medication. Double-blind refers to conditions where

the individuals in the trial and those administering the drugs do not know what is active medication and what is placebo.

I would like to bring your attention to an article published in the Lancet, January 12 1980, the vaccine reviewed was the BCG, (immunisation against tuberculosis). It reported that though the protective efficacy of BCG, was not rigorously assessed, this BCG was increasingly used in Europe during the 1920's.

From 1935 to 1955 the first well controlled trials of BCG were organised only after a serious accident in the production of the BCG vaccine had left 72 children dead from tuberculosis within a few months of inoculation. Of these trials, the Lancet goes on to comment that, "their results varied strikingly and mysteriously", from 0% to 80% effectiveness. (Note the results of the above measles vaccine studies on childhood mortality varying from little more than 0% to 90%). Consequently in the 1970's, the largest controlled field trial ever done on the BCG vaccine, was organised, with 260,000 participants, comparing equal sized vaccine and placebo control groups. Not only did the results show NO evidence of a protective effect but slightly more tuberculosis cases have appeared in vaccinated than in equal sized placebo control (non-vaccinated) groups.

As a consequence of this trial, the BCG vaccine was continued to be used. It appears as though evidence of its ineffectiveness had made no difference whatsoever.

Most of the previous BCG studies were unable to establish the ineffectiveness of the BCG vaccine. Assuming there was no intention to falsify results, this must have been due to the inadequacies of the trials. Trials that did not take into account other factors, for example:

- ➢ Comparing groups that were not strictly comparable.
- ➢ Inconsistencies in disease classification, between groups and also inconsistencies before and after vaccination.
- ➢ Inaccuracies in diagnosis.
- ➢ Studies may not have taken into account natural declines in disease rate that generally occur when other living conditions improve.

> ➤ When deciding whether to vaccinate against measles we appear to have a similar situation. The above trials in developing countries have specifically admitted to not having strictly comparable groups of vaccinated and non-vaccinated. They also warn of the dangers of allying those results to situations in the developed countries i.e. the UK. One study shows quite graphically the impact of improved living conditions on mortality.

Certainly there are no studies with double-blind placebo-controlled trials. What would be the results of such a trial on measles vaccination?

It has been mentioned that placebo-controlled trials would be unethical now. This does not explain why they were not carried out in the first place. Dr Clements states that the measles vaccines were introduced when there was no alternative to measles epidemics. In the UK over 95% reduction in mortality had occurred BEFORE the introduction of measles vaccine. This is undoubtedly due' to aspects of increased standards of living, a point that is further demonstrated by the results of the Tahiti study referenced by Dr Clements.

There are in fact many primary health care measures and conditions of diet and life-style that have had a dramatic effect on measles mortality, unfortunately these factors are overlooked by drug companies which leads to statements where one feels the only measures available are drugs, i.e. vaccines, which is of course not true.

We therefore have a situation where it is difficult to assess the impact of measles vaccination especially in a developed country, such as the UK, where few, if any, adequate trials have been carried out. We also have to consider the possible effects of the vaccine.

With regard to safety Dr Clements states that, "As far as adverse events are concerned, a placebo group is not necessary because one can measure the frequency of a given sign or symptom in the general population and compare that rate to the same sign or symptom in vaccine recipients." This is sufficient for comparing risk of adverse effects of a new measles vaccine with the risks of an existing vaccine, but does not give any indication of the risks of the present vaccine compared to not being vaccinated.

When there was an opportunity to conduct safety and efficacy trials comparing vaccinated and non-vaccinated, vaccine producers chose not to carry these out. We know that many studies are from developing countries and with regard to safety we see that studies have been grossly inadequate. As late as 1975 in the Transactions of The Royal Society of Tropical Medicine (R.G.Hendrickse) it is stated "No figures (of vaccine risk) are available from developing countries". This is not to be confused with there being no risk, but that the risk cannot be assessed because "No figures are available..."

To illustrate this point further, the US National Academy of Sciences published a report in Sept 1993 in which the American Academy of paediatrics reaffirmed "its long standing position that the benefits of immunisation far outweigh the risks". However, Russell Alexander, a panel member and professor of epidemiology at the University of Washington, says he is disappointed that the panel did not compare the risk of vaccination with the risks of going unvaccinated!

How was it therefore possible to come to the conclusion that the benefits of immunisation outweigh the risks when there was no comparison with unimmunised? The benefit of a procedure is a statement of advantage over another procedure, or the advantage over not carrying out the procedure at all. Since there was no comparison of immunisation with another procedure, or with being unimmunised, the conclusions of the American Academy of Paediatrics are not based on scientific reasoning and are almost meaningless. Their position only serves to illustrate the prejudice that exists within many of those interested in promoting vaccines.

Studies now emerging do in fact link measles vaccination with adverse effects. For example Crohn's Disease, an inflammatory bowel disorder, with associated pain, digestive disturbances and joint abnormalities. (The Lancet vol.345 April 29 1995). This can be a serious disease and may take years to develop fully, but can start in childhood with digestive disturbances and consequently developmental problems.

As stated by the manufacturers of measles vaccine, adverse effects include:
…fever, rash, conjunctivitis, coryza, pharyngitis, bronchitis, convulsions, encephalitis, thrombocytopenic purpura and even death.

There are many difficulties to overcome, in obtaining an accurate answer to the question of 'vaccine damage risk' i.e. the real frequency of adverse effects. Firstly, the sources of data for adverse reactions are obtained from orthodox medical doctors notifying the health authorities and the relevant pharmaceutical companies.

Many doctors admit, and it is generally accepted, that the number of adverse reactions reported are an underestimate of the true value. Official experts readily acknowledge that this is partly because they are unsure of the reactions and partly because they do not want to report an accident they feel they may have caused.

It is interesting to note, that in countries where reporting is compulsory, the number of adverse effects to vaccines are higher than those where reporting is voluntary (UK). In the UK doctors are 'asked' to report adverse reactions, but there is no formal requirement to do so.

In the UK the situation has also been recently made worse by the additional factor of financial incentives for doctors, to encourage them to achieve the highest possible immunisation 'targets'. This means that doctors, who vaccinate the largest percentage of patients on their books, stand to gain the most. Whilst those who exercise greater discretion in the administration of vaccines, due to adverse reaction or because they are willing to support parents who do not wish their children to be immunised, are financially penalised.

There are also certain time restraints placed on the appearance of symptoms, if they are to be attributed to the vaccine. For example, symptoms of adverse reactions must be apparent in an individual within 72 hours for the whooping cough vaccine and 8-20 days for the live vaccines of measles, mumps, rubella and polio.

However, just as it may take many years to die of a serious disease, of which there may have been no apparent symptoms in the early stages, it may take equally as long for the effects of medical procedures to manifest as recognisable disease symptoms. There are therefore obvious drawbacks to such strict time restrictions.

The withdrawal of the Urabe strain of mumps virus used in MMR vaccine illustrates quite clearly the phenomena of under-reporting with regard to adverse effects. The Urabe strain was thought to be linked to meningitis because the vaccine virus particles were isolated from the cerebrospinal fluid of affected children. Canada stopped using the vaccine in 1989. In the UK however, where alternative strains of mumps vaccine were not so readily available, various studies were conducted to assess the risk.

Studies based on voluntary reports gave reassuringly low estimates, one case of meningitis per 143,000 (notification by doctors) to 250,000 (voluntary reports by paediatricians). But when greater efforts were made to identify cases, for instance by cross-linking laboratory and hospital reports to vaccination records, the risk rose to between 1 in 4,000 and 1 in 21,000. These findings suggested significant under-reporting of Urabe vaccine-associated meningitis, and led to the withdrawal of the vaccine from the market in 1992. (*Parliamentary office of science and technology, "Vaccines and their future role in public health",July 1995. Also Dawbarns, solicitors, Kings Lynn, MMR & MR factsheet*).

The benefit of immunisation is further diminished when we consider the duration of apparent immunity. Vaccine immunity is not as long lasting as that from the naturally acquired disease, we shall look at two consequences of this.

Firstly as immunity diminishes in adulthood there may be a delayed susceptibility to measles at an older age. Symptoms of which are generally more debilitating, with complications being more frequent and more difficult to treat than the natural childhood disease at the normal age.

In addition, as immunity diminishes in adulthood, vaccinated mothers have less immunity to pass on to their children than those that have contracted the disease naturally. Thus we see an increase in the number of measles cases in young babies where the risk of adverse effects are increased. Whereas children would normally be protected for the first year or so if maternal immunity had been acquired naturally.

It may therefore be necessary to give booster shots throughout life, in which case risk assessments will need to evaluate multiple immunisations over a longer period of time.
Therefore the question of the benefit of measles vaccine compared to the risk, in developing countries, can hardly be answered by reference to the studies given to date. The question is even more difficult to assess in developed countries such as the UK where it seems that we are assessing a questionable benefit compared to an unknown risk.

Perhaps the most interesting point of discussion comes from Dr Clements response to the question of ". . . the benefit of eradicating measles in the average child in the UK." Dr Clements states "By definition if measles is eradicated, the child is unlikely to get measles. So he or she will not develop complications or die from a disease he or she never gets. We are talking about the absence of a disease resulting in a reduced disease burden." He goes on to say... "How do fences around electricity pylons improve the health of children?" He continues... "Answer, they don't, they reduce the chances of children touching or climbing on them and getting killed."

The analogy is a wonderful example of the thinking behind much orthodox medical treatment including that of immunisation. Firstly there is an assumption that the symptoms of measles have a wholly negative effect in the individual. I shall look at various examples including that of measles to see how this interpretation may be false.

A method of interpreting symptoms developed by Dr Randolphe Nesse, practising physician, Professor of Academic Affairs in the Department of Psychiatry, University of Michigan School of Medicine, and Dr George Williams, professor Emeritus of Ecology and Evolution at the State University of New York, member of the US National Academy of Science, has given rise to the term 'Darwinian medicine'. The concept although claimed to be new, has in fact been used by complementary therapists for centuries.

The basis of their rationale comes from acknowledging the fact that many symptoms are produced in order to maintain the health of the individual. The symptoms will, therefore, depend on the particular susceptibility of the individual and the conditions that the individual is currently subjected to. The term Darwinian medicine relates to the hypothesis that these symptoms have therefore evolved for the survival of that species and individual.

That is, the symptoms have a purpose, they are not merely malfunctions. Examples given are; the beneficial response of fever in combating micro-organisms during an infection; the role of diarrhoea in the evacuation of patheogenic organisms; the removal of iron from blood circulation in early bacterial infection appears as anaemia, this results in the decrease of the iron supply to the bacteria, which does not allow the bacteria to flourish; accompanied swelling when spraining a joint to stop motion and increase in scavenger cells to remove damaged tissue; morning sickness and its role in protecting the foetus from toxins.

The possible suppression of symptoms without understanding the larger context of their function may therefore lead to more serious consequences.
For example "Fever has only recently been revealed (*by the orthodox medical establishment*) as a beneficial response to infection. The response is triggered by bacterial toxins, and the resulting increase in body temperature is hostile to invading microorganisms. Reduce the fever - using aspirin, for instance -and the disease may last longer, as Timothy Doran of Johns Hopkins University, Baltimore, has recently demonstrated in the case of chickenpox. "(New Scientist, 23-10-93). My italics.

After contracting measles and other childhood illnesses (e.g.. chickenpox, scarlet fever, whooping cough, rubella, mumps and may be others), it has been widely accepted by many health practitioners, including experienced orthodox paediatricians that this is often beneficial for the general health of many children. Specifically it has been shown that children contracting measles naturally were less likely to suffer from allergic conditions such as asthma, eczema and hayfever, (Lancer June 29 1996).

The effects of symptoms and illnesses may have consequences way beyond that of the acute problems immediately following a disease. For example, The Lancet 5 Jan 1985, reports on a study investigating the phenomenon of measles virus infection without the appearance of typical measles rash. The presence of measles antibodies in individuals is evidence of measles virus infection, however some do not produce the typical measles rash. In adulthood, (average age in the study was 38 years), for those with antibodies but NO rash, there was shown to be an increased incidence of immunoreactive diseases, sebaceous skin diseases, degenerative diseases of bone and cartilage, and certain tumours.

The report concludes that, at the time of infection, it may be dangerous to interfere with the immune response by administering a passive immunisation. It also states that "the absence of a rash may imply that intracellular virus escapes neutralisation during the acute infection and this, in turn, might give rise to the development of diseases subsequently".

The report does not question the implications of active viral immunisation where, of course, specific antibodies are produced without the appearance of typical measles rash. In addition we have no means of assessing this since we do not have studies that compare immunised with unimmunised.

It has been possible to demonstrate the benefit, in overall and long term health, of having certain types of disease symptomology. But can we show any negative effects of suppression of disease using vaccines?

Dr Michel Odent at The Primal Health research centre in London published a report in the Journal of the American Medical Association showing how the whooping cough vaccine increases the incidence of asthma by 5 to 6 times in those vaccinated compared to those unvaccinated. It appears as though the vaccine creates a chronic lung weakness in the form of asthma, whereas children that have been allowed to overcome whooping cough naturally may be strengthened in this area.

Therefore, in order to assess the benefit of a medical procedure, we need to observe its total affect on the health of the individual, over a sufficiently long period of time. Healthy individuals may not have symptoms of illness, for example, healthy individuals do not have raised temperatures, but they are capable of producing a raised temperature under certain conditions i.e. a fever, a very necessary response when dealing with an infection. There is a difference between a healthy individual not needing to create a fever and an individual unable to create a fever, the latter being the far unhealthier option.

It has been found that death rates increase in patients who are less able to produce a sufficiently high fever in response to infections (American Journal of Medicine. 68:344-355, 1980).

By eradicating measles with vaccination we are not necessarily creating healthy individuals, but perhaps suppressing symptoms thus producing individuals incapable of producing certain types of inflammatory reactions. Dr Clements response to the question of the benefit of eradicating measles does not take this into account. It is not necessarily the case that an individual without certain disease symptomology is necessarily healthier than an individual with those symptoms.

Dr Clements does acknowledge this. However, his analogy…
"How do fences around electricity pylons improve the health of children? Answer, they don't, they reduce the chances of children touching or climbing on them and getting killed."
…serves to illustrate the limited medical understanding with regard to the effects of vaccination and disease symptoms.

That is, measles cannot be analogous to an electricity pylon, i.e. a wholly negative burden. Previous medical practitioners have, removed tonsils, removed adenoids, suppressed symptoms of fever, etc., essentially interpreted the various parts and responses as unnecessary burdens and have later learned this to be not true.

The fence cannot be analogous to immunisation, as immunisation has consequences that affect the health of individuals. The fence may be more dangerous than what it is supposedly guarding. In addition we are learning that the act of guarding, (suppressing), can also be detrimental for overall and long term health.

We have then to face an additional question as to the value of immunisation compared to alternatives. Given that there may be a possible value in being able to display certain symptoms under given conditions. It seems likely that another way to avoid problems from measles, or any other illness, is to avoid the conditions that give rise to them and raise the level of health of individuals in order to overcome future problems effectively.

None of the references have made any comparison to alternatives. One study does show the dramatic impact of improved living conditions on reducing mortality. Similarly UK statistics show a 95% reduction in measles mortality before the introduction of measles vaccination.

Dr Clements states "I do not know of a legitimate public health measure which could be administered and which could have a similar effect to vaccination in reducing disease incidence".

Again this serves to highlight the lack of interest in methods other than pharmaceutical. For example Vitamin A supplementation has been shown to reduce the mortality rate due to measles, in under 2 year olds, by seven times. (BMJ, 1987, 294). Many studies show increase eye problems and deaths in children with vitamin A deficiency. How would immunisation compare with vitamin A supplementation? Unfortunately we do not know. Finally, to illustrate the unstable nature of what we 'know' about vaccines; in the UK travellers are now advised by immunisation clinics that there is not an effective cholera vaccine. Dr Clements seems to disagree; in that this relates to emergency situations and that the problem is the amount of time needed to create an antibody response to the vaccine (two weeks).

"As a result the WHO recommends that in these emergency situations, the first line of defence should be providing safe clean water and proper waste disposal".

Which ever view we take, a strong criticism still exists and that is:

- ➢ The numbers of individuals that were given the vaccine with the impression that it was effective.
- ➢ The amount of time taken to establish this fact.
- ➢ The inadequacy of the initial trials in not establishing the ineffectiveness of the vaccine.
- ➢ The relative importance of alternatives, i.e. safe clean water and proper waste disposal.

Dr Clements, given the above response to the details we have received from yourself on behalf of the WHO, are we to believe that we have established the safety and effectiveness of other vaccines compared to safer alternatives?

I very much thank you for your time in this matter and in anticipation of your response. There are very many people that have appreciated your comments such that we have been able to debate these issues publicly.

Yours sincerely
Trevor Gunn
For The Informed Parent